Tales of a Forensic Pathologist

Also by Zoya Schmuter:

- From Russia with Luck
- We Borrowed Grandchildren for Swiss Vacation

Tales of a Forensic Pathologist

Zoya Schmuter, MD

iUniverse, Inc.
New York   Bloomington

Tales of a Forensic Pathologist

Copyright © 2009 by Zoya Schmuter, M.D.

*All rights reserved. No part of this book may be used or reproduced by
any means, graphic, electronic, or mechanical, including photocopying,
recording, taping or by any information storage retrieval system
without the written permission of the publisher except in the case
of brief quotations embodied in critical articles and reviews.*

*The identities of people involved in the forensic cases are fictional Any
similarities are coincidental.*

iUniverse books may be ordered through booksellers or by contacting:

iUniverse
1663 Liberty Drive
Bloomington, IN 47403
www.iuniverse.com
1-800-Authors (1-800-288-4677)

*Because of the dynamic nature of the Internet, any Web addresses or links
contained in this book may have changed since publication and may no
longer be valid. The views expressed in this work are solely those of the
author and do not necessarily reflect the views of the publisher, and the
publisher hereby disclaims any responsibility for them.*

ISBN: 978-1-4401-2676-5 (pbk)
ISBN: 978-1-4401-2677-2 (ebk)

Printed in the United States of America

iUniverse rev. date: 2/24/2009

Contents

INTRODUCTION

I am a medical doctor—a pathologist. As of the moment of this writing, I have just retired. For the last twenty-two years, I have worked as a Medical Examiner Level II (that is, a senior) in the Office of Chief Medical Examiner (OCME) of New York. Over the years, I performed thousands of autopsies and testified in courts hundreds of times. Many of these cases, in my mind, present interest for a general reader, especially given the attention to our profession in the last decade. I always thought of publishing selected stories, saving some materials and writing fragments. I periodically gave students a lecture on "Challenging Cases in Forensic Pathology."

The stories in this book are based on real cases, but some details have been changed or added. One reason is that, as many years passed, time played one or two tricks with my memory, erasing some details. More importantly, there was no point in revealing identities of the involved people. In fact, I went to great length to avoid this. Any similarities are just coincidental.

My book describes the experiences of a medical examiner. This unique profession is a frequent subject of movies, TV shows, and fiction books, which mystify and fascinate the public in spite of brutal reality. I am aware, in fact, that this is not the first book in this field, but I think that this is one of very few that describes the broad and complicated medical range of our profession.

The truth is that homicide covers fewer than 15% of all cases performed by medical examiners. My non-fiction book creates public awareness of some important issues of our life beyond the homicides such as drug intoxication deaths, child abuse and negligence, the sudden death of young people, the importance of timely diagnostics, the prophylactics of sudden infant deaths, and the need for attentiveness to rare diseases. On family or hospital requests, we, as part of independent objective organizations, deal with numerous hospital cases, work with clinicians, go in depth into laboratory studies, hospital charts, literature searches, conferences, and consultations with specialized experts in order to understand the cause of death. This is very important for the family, but it is equally important for the physicians for the best management of future patients and analysis of possible mistakes. I hope that the cases in this book, selected from my personal experience, shed the light on and do justice to our profession.

In order to lay the foundation on which the stories are based, in the first part of the book, I am giving a memoir of my first years in the New York office, opening a window to the background of my life and work in one of the largest and best offices in the world.

I graduated from medical school in the former Soviet Union and worked there as a pediatrician and later as an anatomic pathologist until 1975. I then was licensed and worked in Israel as a pathologist. I start these stories from my move to New York from Detroit, Michigan, where, as a foreign graduate, I went through the process of re-training and licensing. I did a four-year residency in anatomic and clinical pathology and an additional year of fellowship in forensic pathology in the Detroit Office of Medical Examiner. Detroit's was a very busy office—after all, not long ago it became infamous by its dubious reputation as the murder capital.

PART 1
I AM A MEDICAL EXAMINER IN NEW YORK

FIRST YEARS

Back in 1986, I started my new job as a medical examiner for the New York Office of the Chief Medical Examiner. Sam, my husband, brought me, along with the necessary furniture, to New York in a van he borrowed at work. Sam was left temporarily behind with the Ford Motor Company, and my son Leonid, 27, with General Motors, and another son Gene, 20, at the University of Michigan. I left behind my first house with my "dream come true" rose garden, magnolia trees around the house, and the creek on the property. I "kissed good-bye" another family member, our Doberman Gingi, who watched me leaving with his sad eyes. And the few friends that we made during our years in Michigan were also left behind. This was my "emigration" from the state of Michigan to the state of New York!

For the time being, I was alone in a small studio in an excellent neighborhood of the Upper East Side. The charming Gracie Mansion with its park and the lovely Finley Walk along the bank of the East River were always here for me, still as irresistible as they were from the first look. I felt in New York as a fish in the water from the moment that I came to this beautiful city. I was forty-nine and starting a new professional life, this time as a medical examiner. I was very grateful to Dr. Werner Spitz, who during my last year of fellowship training in forensic pathology, gave me confidence and respect for myself and this new profession. And here I was in this huge city, in a big, prestigious office with all new people, and alone in my studio on the East River.

The Office of the Chief Medical Examiner (OCME), in

addition to the Manhattan branch also included offices in Brooklyn and Queens, which I was not aware of at the time of my interview. There were about thirty medical doctors, forensic pathologists, among some 300 other employees, all belonging to the City Health Department. It was very different from the Detroit office, which was small and had only a few doctors. Detroit had one and a half histology positions, a toxicology lab with five specialists; and two police investigators. The office was quite poorly equipped. Autopsy reports were handwritten on standard forms.

The New York office was a huge Institute of Pathology for the entire city. Many hospitals in New York City were doing everything possible to avoid autopsies. Why? Is it because the autopsies are not as profitable as biopsies? As a result, my new place of employment was overloaded and not only with victims of homicide, accident, suicide, and natural death at home, but we also had the complicated hospital cases that challenge any highly skilled pathologist.

It was extremely difficult physically yet exciting and interesting to work in this unusual office. The excellent staff of the histology lab, led by a very pleasant and relatively young black woman named Beverly, probably did not realize themselves how professional and efficient they were. Several years later the histology staff was further enhanced and expanded with more personnel and extended to the whole floor. The unbelievable speed of response they showed in delivering microscopy slides would beat the speed of many hospital laboratories. The toxicology laboratory, headed by a tall, good-looking Ph.D. named Marina S., of Yugoslavian origin, had a large staff and offered multiple analyses. They didn't deliver the results nearly as fast as histology, taking three to six months to respond. But after ten years with the new Chief Medical Examiner, toxicology response and reporting were drastically improved after modernizing and updating to a new state-of-the-art facility.

When I went to work for the New York office, among the

total of thirty doctors in all the branches, at least five or six were Russian doctors, and all of us worked in the Manhattan office. That made us a quite visible third of the Manhattan staff. This was a bit of a surprise for me; in Detroit I was the only Russian doctor in my department at William Beaumont Hospital and also in the Detroit Office of Medical Examiners. To be honest, I was not pleased by this Russian "invasion," because I soon discovered that they spoke only Russian among themselves, and I began to worry that my English might disappear instead of constantly improving. My attempts to speak English with the others were met with hostility.

Our boss and his two female deputies were all American born, while most of the doctors under them were of foreign origin. It was strange but I soon understood the reason: we were greatly overworked and largely underpaid. The boss and the deputies did not participate in sharing the big load of autopsies. That was different from the way it was in Detroit, where Dr. Spitz and all his deputies were actively involved in carrying the workload. For the relatively young deputies such an arrangement definitely did not improve either their experience or confidence. Our boss at that time had serious legal and media problems caused by his interpretation of a "famous " public case involving police brutality; so he definitely wasn't looking for more troubles. The troubles came anyway, after he left the New York Office. I was saddened by that, because he was a good man and a good forensic pathologist, but perhaps he was not suited to be a political appointee.

Later in 1990, with the appointment of the new chief, Dr. Hirsch, when the workload diminished (still on the high end compared to that of other offices but definitely becoming more reasonable), and the salary improved, American doctors replaced most of the others. But before that happened we really worked heroically, no complaints, because we were survivors without many choices; we just did what we were supposed to do, which was to work very hard.

Actually all the work in Manhattan was done by five or six people. Every day I had three to five autopsies plus external examinations. During my first year I had 600 cases! For comparison, the average caseload in later years was 250. And the cases we had were really difficult, especially considering that it was my first year as attending forensic pathologist. Soon the physically hard work caused tendonitis in my right hand, but I stoically hid it from everybody. After all, "never complain" was a slogan of the American society. I never went to see an orthopedist because over the telephone I was informed that I had to pay 300 dollars for an immediate appointment, and I was not sure what insurance coverage I had. I also had negative feelings toward the doctor's office when the receptionist asked for my coverage and money before the doctor had even seen me. I was still new to the world of the American health care system.

As I mentioned, our boss was in the middle of a big problem with one autopsy that had been performed a few years earlier, and I had read about it when I was still in Detroit. But I did not know the essence of the case, and at my new job people never discussed this sensitive issue (at least not with me). As I learned during all these many years the atmosphere was always very cautious, and people kept away from rumors or even jokes about the boss, the deputies, and office problems. Back in the Soviet Union we were afraid to discuss political issues, fearing for dear life; but we could however criticize our coworkers without fear of losing our jobs for that. But here people were visibly fearful, untrusting, and very competitive at work. I talked to Sam about this; he thought that smaller companies were even more inclined to have these kinds of problems.

The Office of the Medical Examiner was never closed; we worked seven days a week. In addition to our busy daily work, management decided to put us on rotation as medical investigators. This duty had previously belonged to other medical personnel or "moonlighting" doctors. But one of the deputies had the "good idea" to save money for the Health Department by replacing the medical investigators with medical examiners, of course without additional wages. The only "strange" thing was that she did not participate in this duty herself. It was a time-consuming job, requiring driving in a car around the whole city often in terrible traffic, going to crime scenes, often in dangerous and strange places.

This deputy usually took upon herself the distribution of cases and personally supervised the drug overdose cases, which were done by the per-diem staffers; and she usually avoided taking on complicated cases. I remember one Sunday when I was extremely busy performing four difficult autopsies, two of them homicides with multiple gunshot wounds. This deputy asked me to work that evening's medical investigator tour in place of somebody who had not shown up for work. I was so tired that I could hardly stand up after such a hard day when she came up with her directive. She did not even consider herself for this task because she knew that the Russian emigrant doctor, only recently hired by this office, would not dare to refuse. Sam left for Detroit without seeing me that Sunday.

On another occasion, late in the summer of 1986, this deputy gave a high-profile case to the fellow-in-training who had been working in the program for only two months. This was the case of the Central Park homicide, later known as the "preppy case," which involved asphyxia by strangulation; apparently she was afraid to perform this autopsy herself. Fortunately for the case and the Office, the fellow, a smart Filipino, Doctor A., did a good job and the prosecutor won the case. Ironically, after a few years this doctor got the job of deputy, when under the newly appointed chief the former deputy left.

It would have been difficult if not impossible to survive at this job at that time if I did not like my work. I was really interested in my new field. I often thought about writing a book, perhaps in the future, "Notes of a Forensic Pathologist." After my experience as a pathologist in the Soviet Union and Israel, the forensic pathology was a fresh field, and my previous experience in pathology was a big plus. On the other hand, I had to deal with the forensic aspects of pathology, with the police with their valuable and mandatory information, and with the legal system of multiple lawyers, prosecutors and defense, hospital doctors, and the relatives of the deceased with their pain and demands. Thank God, we did not have to deal with the New York press. We had the services of our own press contact and public relations person. She, a very nice person, is still there, having survived three bosses, and dealing on a daily basis with the media under the careful watch of the Chief Medical Examiner.

After seven months in Manhattan I was sent to work in the Brooklyn branch office, with morgue technicians and facilities that were part of Kings County Hospital. The Brooklyn office was a new world for me, requiring a long daily drive from 79th Street in Manhattan to the Kings County Hospital in Brooklyn. The poor Brooklyn facility had two rooms for doctors, the autopsy room and the restroom in the basement, which was quite dangerous to use due to the possibility of intrusion from outside. Also, there was the clerk's room, the police room, and the deputy's room on the second floor. The rooms in the basement did not have a telephone, so important in our work, and for every telephone call we had to run upstairs.

The morgue technicians belonged to the hospital staff, not to the Office of the Medical Examiner, and it was very important to have a good relationship with them if we wanted to have their vital help. Fortunately for me they accepted me as "their own," perhaps because of my Russian accent, which may have appealed to their sense of solidarity, as a part of the "second class" office, at least in the eyes of the Manhattan management. I had by now enough experience in autopsies so they immediately appreciated how efficient I was. The telephone problem was a serious one, and I decided to do something about it; surprisingly it did not bother the rest of the "basement" doctors who came from Haiti and the Philippines and were not spoiled by convenient telephone service. But already being in this country for nine years, I thought the inconvenience was unacceptable. Every morning before starting work I would go to the hospital administrator for a few minutes to bother him about the telephone issue. Finally we were successful and the doctors received their telephone. I enjoyed the victory but not the convenience of having the telephone because I was soon and unexpectedly transferred back to Manhattan.

My return coincided with changes in the position of Chief Medical Examiner. After a brief search by the Department of Health, the mayor appointed a new boss, Dr. Hirsch. It was the winter of 1989; the new era in the OCME had begun.

I LOVE NEW YORK

Meanwhile, life continued. I was in love with New York from the moment I first got here. The city was alive and upbeat and did not look that huge to me. In my mind I saw Manhattan as it was on the subway map, with its well-organized parallel streets and avenues and its excellent public transportation system. Never in my life had I seen such a variety of people with different languages and customs. In general, I found New Yorkers very friendly with plenty of common sense and a good attitude toward life and people. In Detroit everyone seemed to be "car people" with meaningless smiles, suburban people with only local interests. In New York I loved walking along the streets and avenues of Manhattan, looking at countless windows of stores and restaurants and people who did not stop to amaze me. After my very uneasy workday I usually walked from our office on the East 30th Street along First Avenue up to East 81st Street, some forty-five minutes, during which my tiredness and irritation would disappear. I thought how lucky I was to be in the USA, to be a medical doctor in this country, to live in New York, to see what I saw, to be healthy, to have my family happy and busy with whatever they were doing.

One of the things that amazed me in New York was the New York dogs, which often resembled their owners. I thought of these dogs as a special tribe that had developed survival skills in this multimillion city. Of course, I missed my red Doberman, Gingi, who was with Sam in Michigan, but our Gingi could learn a thing or two from the dogs of New York. Their owners would often leave them tied to a tree or a pole and disappear inside a store or a restaurant for an indefinite time. And these poor New Yorkers, the dogs of different breed, age, height, and looks, just stood there looking through the entrance with sadness, dedication, and love on their faces, waiting for their owners and not paying attention to the traffic, people, and any offerings of affection to them. "I belong only to my beloved owner. He will come now and we will be united again" was written on these dogs' faces. These New York dogs would never do what our Gingi once did when I was talking with one of our Michigan neighbors. Gingi probably got tired of our long conversation; he put his posterior leg up and made "pee-pee" on my acquaintance. But at the beginning of my New York life, seeing the faces of the dogs and feeling their fear to be abundant, I sometimes looked for their owners inside the store. Unfortunately, the dogs could not give me their owner's description, and my test for the similarity between dogs and their owners didn't always work. At that time I felt dogs' pain more sharply because I was lonely in this big city.

In my studio I had a tiny kitchen, but I did not cook much for myself even though I am a good cook. On my way home from the office, usually after 6pm, I often bought half a deliciously grilled chicken, with Greek salad, fresh bread, fruits and, of course, my favorite Italian grapes at Edik's, a small grocery store on First Avenue and 81st Street. I usually bought all other supplies at Associated, the supermarket across the street from Edik's. It was amazing how in such a big city we all got stuck with the same few neighborhood food stores and the few people working there, and they knew us and we knew them for already ten or fifteen years. In my mind the short man with black mustache was Eddie (Edik in Russian), the Greek. I have now been living in the same neighborhood for over twenty years, just in gradually improved apartments, and Edik's was still there yesterday.

On 86th Street between First and Second Avenue was the restaurant where Sam and I would frequently go, the German one, but all the dishes there were like the Russian dishes that I myself could prepare. They were like the ones served in my mother's house as well as in mine: schnitzel with cabbage (I serve schnitzel with mashed potatoes), potato latkes with applesauce (we serve them with sour cream). In the complicated history of Russia many things were intermixed with things from German culture, even tsars and their traditionally German wives. In fact, even in medicine the German textbooks and authors were ahead of the American, at least in the first half of the twentieth century. Of course, after WWII the German language nearly disappeared as a foreign language from schools in favor of English, and American professional literature started to dominate the main references. But culinary customs were apparently much stronger, as I discovered in New York.

Sam was also in love with New York. Every weekend or at least every other weekend he was flying from Detroit to New York, spending hours on flight, arrivals, departures, delays, and driving to and from airports. He missed me in Detroit as I missed him in New York. Often I called him at night. "You are homeless," he told me once, because it was difficult to catch me during the day. The reason for this was my busy life and also claustrophobia that I felt in this small studio with the tiny kitchen after my spacious and beautiful Michigan home with its huge kitchen and cozy dining room near a bay window overlooking magnolia trees and a stream in the ravine. Well, Sam had successfully sold this house, luckily the market improved in a timely way for us, and he temporarily moved to an apartment. It had been difficult for him to find an apartment because most of the owners did not like our dog Gingi as much as we did. On some of Sam's trips to New York I barely saw him because every other weekend I worked Saturday and Sunday.

Soon my son Leonid joined me in New York after getting a job with Merrill Lynch. He rented a large studio-apartment in a brownstone building, classy outside and ugly inside, on the West Side, with me being his guarantor. His first impression after living in the Motor City was that New Yorkers stayed too close to each other and there was no space, but he soon became one of the many New Yorkers who enjoyed its variety of foods and unique cultural life.

A half year after my move, Sam moved in with the remainder of our furniture and Gingi. Sam had sold our house, found a new job with a high-tech company on Long Island, lost nine years toward his Ford Motor Company pension, and came happily to join us in New York. Gingi embraced New York with all his heart; he immediately became a real "city boy," joining the army of the East Side dogs, every morning and evening strolling with us through the Carl Shurz Park in the fresh air from the East River, the spring red, blue, and white tulips that he loved to smell replacing his love for my Michigan roses, and the green lawns that he was using as a run.

Sam easily adapted without complaint to my small studio, and so did the dog. Our one regret was that we missed buying the one-bedroom apartment with an astonishing view on the fifteenth floor of the 10 East End building. This apartment was not large, but it had huge windows which displayed the beauty of the East River and a partial view of Carl Shurz Park. When I first saw the apartment, I wondered how one could live there: I had a feeling that I would be suspended in a completely open space in the middle of the city. We hesitated to buy it because at that time Sam still had not finalized the job in New York. So, our hesitation lasted too long; somebody came, looked at this apartment, and bought it for cash. But we did not dwell on that for long; we bought in the same building a not-so-fascinating one-bedroom with no view. But it was less expensive and good enough for the two of us and Gingi.

Early every morning Sam commuted fifty-five miles to Long Island. He alternated driving with a new coworker, so that the one who wasn't driving had a chance to get a little more sleep. But Sam had to really watch his new absentminded friend, a Ph.D. and former colonel of Iranian navy. One time when Sam opened his eyes from the passenger seat, his friend was also sleeping in the driver's seat while the car was idling at a green traffic light. On another occasion, his friend drove away with Sam's bag after letting Sam out of the car, and Sam had to run after the car — to no avail. More than once Sam would wait at 6am at the doorway of our building for his friend to pick him up, while his friend was doing the same thing at his building, confused about whose turn it was. Once his car ran out of gas in the middle of a long stretch of the Long Island Expressway near exit 39. They had to climb a high slope through wild thorn bushes before they could get to a gas station. Otherwise, Sam was doing really well at this new place, developing robots and often going to Detroit on business.

After graduating from the University of Michigan in Ann Arbor our younger son Gene found a job with the Grumman Aerospace Corporation on Long Island. He rented an apartment in Queens, we bought him a car, and now all my family were united within the New York boroughs, in three different one-bedrooms. Gingi stayed with Sam and me. I guess we all settled for life in New York. And it looked like I was going to make it through the "boot camp" of mine.

***

To get to Brooklyn I drove the used car that Gene brought for me from Detroit, the same car he used to move in with his stuff. Without that car I would have had to spend three hours a day on the subway. In addition, the Kings County Hospital area and the nearby subway were not safe places in 1988. Once returning after my late hours at work I found myself in the middle of a nest of violent teenagers arguing with each other on the subway platform. Luckily for me no guns were pulled. Another time, returning late after a busy day on Christmas Eve, I was in an empty subway car with only one other woman when a young man of suspicious appearance suddenly appeared in front of us asking for money. Nothing happened; after giving him the small amount of money that we had, the woman and I escaped to another car with more passengers in it. Actually this was my first unpleasant encounter in New York. So thanks to my son, I started using a car to get to Brooklyn.

One day I locked my keys inside the running car near Kings County Hospital. Naturally I went to the nearby driving school to ask for help. Nobody there could help me, and I was thinking about calling the police when a black man who was driving by offered to help me for five dollars. Of course, I agreed and in front of my eyes he almost immediately unlocked my car door with a long wire that he got from his car. I was amazed: no car could withstand his desire to get in.

On another occasion, Sam was driving and I was in the passenger seat. While waiting for a red light to change, a pedestrian started pointing to our right front tire. Sam asked what the matter was, and this street-smart guy said that he saw a nail in the tire. He kneeled near the wheel and directed Sam to move slightly back so that the nail would become more visible. When Sam got out of the car, he saw (surprise-surprise) two nails sticking out of the tire. "Luckily" the guy had with him the required tool for pulling out the nails and rubber sealant to fill the nail holes. He claimed he was coming home from work at a tire shop. To take out the two nails he charged only $20. The entire business took less than three minutes. The whole trick of holding the nails between his two fingers under the slowly reversing tire until they punctured it soon became evident — but not until after the three minutes needed for the quick fix while we were holding up traffic.

I really think of New York as a safe city, especially considering my wandering around at different hours of the day, sometimes really late. We just have to be alert and exhibit common sense, as in any big city. For many years in New York I did not have any personally dangerous encounters. Having stated that, I just want to tell about one recent event.

On a beautiful summer day of 2004, my last day before a two-week vacation, I was too relaxed and lost my alertness. I left my open car with the keys in my hand acting as a good citizen to give directions to the driver of a van stopped at the passenger side of my car, a road map extended through its driver's window. I was the victim of a trivial trick when another man from the van opened the driver's door of my car and stole my handbag containing all documents, credit cards, my office badge, my social security card, cell phone, some cash and who knows what else. It happened right near the entrance to the Jewish Community Center where I just finished swimming. Interestingly, the JCC surveillance camera outside the building picked up the whole event, everything, even the license plate on the van. Of course, I reported the incident to the police, who were very good to me (they like medical examiners), but apparently they had more important things to do than chasing my stolen bag. It was a big headache to cancel my cards and replace my IDs. But I was quite surprised after my two-week vacation, when my damaged badge, social security card, driver's license, personalized transportation Metrocard, and even Metropolitan Museum membership card were "found" somewhere in Brooklyn. That was really a New York–style robbery.

Driving home from the Brooklyn office every day, I enjoyed the grand view of the downtown, the Wall Street area, and the World Trade Center Towers, the emblem of New York. I felt so proud living and working here. We all were deeply wounded on September 11, 2001, by the destruction of the Towers and the 3,000 people falling with them. I would like to see something even grander in place of the Twin Towers; but thousands of people were gone, leaving behind their families with the permanent pain in their hearts.

ABOUT OCME

Dr. Charles Hirsch was a tall, lean, and fit man with a voice that made him sound older than he was. I read all his published papers I could find, and I liked what I read. He was of the same good Dr. Fisher's forensic school that my mentor, Dr. Werner Spitz, came from. All his publications were solid and serious. He brought with him couple of young doctors, one of them Dr. Adams, an intelligent and pleasant person with great potential who needed good experience, and another young fellow who started his training with Dr. Hirsch in the Suffolk County office. I was right about the potential of Dr. Adams, who after a few years with us moved on to become the chief medical examiner in Tampa, Florida. With Dr. Hirsch, he published a chapter for the new edition of the Fisher and Spitz forensic pathology textbook. I liked Dr. Adams and respected him, because he really tried to learn by working hard, never avoiding difficult cases.

Speaking of difficult cases, I have always wondered why some people consciously choosing this specialty would try to avoid the difficulties in our profession, or try to become supervisors without first gaining enough experience. They are bound to remain handicapped, probably understand that, but cowardly perpetuate the pattern. Maybe they do not believe in themselves? Dr. Spitz, my former boss and the first forensic pathology teacher, exemplified an absolutely different attitude. Being a highly experienced and widely recognized forensic pathologist, and the author of the primary textbook, he never slowed down, never stopped performing autopsies. Once when I was his fellow I was working on a multiple gunshot wound homicide case, and he came in and immediately solved my confusion about the two-inches-in-diameter round-pattern abrasion on the top of the head. He looked at the body and pointed out to me the exit wound on one foot. "Go to the scene and look from where he fell after being shot," Dr. Spitz suggested. He was right. The victim had first been shot in the apartment, and then, trying to escape, had been shot on the balcony. He had fallen from the balcony onto a two-inch vertical pipe that protruded from the ground. I found his hair inside of this pipe. That was Dr. Spitz! His conferences were always brilliant with fresh new looks at things, products of his sharp brain and eyes. These meetings were also provocative, offering inspiring discussions and encouraging the expression of alternative views. It remained to be seen if my new boss could match Dr. Spitz.

In addition to the new doctors, Dr. Hirsch brought with him a very capable administrator, David Schomburg, who was an excellent manager and initiated many changes to modernize our office. He organized and trained medical investigators to replace the "moonlighters" in going to scenes of investigation, which freed the forensic pathologists to focus on our prime responsibilities. He also led the office into the computer age.

I liked how Dr. Hirsch spoke one-on-one with each of us in order to hear our suggestions for improvements. One suggestion I made was to figure out a way to overcome the unacceptable delay in finalizing "pending cases," that still took more than six months. Relatives had insurance and had to deal with problems of ever-increasing prices for funeral arrangements. In Dr. Spitz's office I was trained not to create unnecessary "pending cases," but it was the frequent pattern for diagnoses in this office. Dr. Hirsch agreed that something needed to be done.

I was really surprised once when Dr. Hirsch, with a hint of tears in his eyes, congratulated me (even hugged me), and told me that he was very proud of me when I passed the Forensic Pathology Board. I must say here, in retrospect, that over years of Dr. Hirsch leadership, the New York Office became one of, if not the, greatest and finest forensic institutions in the world. Many of our fellow-pathologists, after training and gaining experience in our office, eventually became Chiefs of offices across the nation.

So now I had everything that was possible and the maximum necessary for a medical doctor in my new country: ECFMG, Flex, Board Certification in Anatomical Pathology and Forensic Pathology. I also had two years of training in clinical pathology, but I decided against taking this specialty board exam because I did not plan to work in that area. Having the training and current knowledge in the field was definitely an advantage and I used it a lot in my work, for example, when talking with clinicians about hospital cases or when reviewing unbelievably thick hospital charts. The laboratory service was on a very high level in the States, and we all relied heavily on lab data. I had the impression that many of the lab analyses were not necessary, but perhaps they were — and anyway they were good business for the hospitals and for the doctors' offices. Of course, as long as the insurance companies paid, the patients would not be that concerned. I myself had good medical insurance because I worked for the Health Department, where salaries were not so high as in private practice but the benefits were better. I gradually understood and appreciated the important benefits of my position, the pension plan, the deferred compensation plan, and the unique doctors' union, which existed only in New York — probably because New York was the most democratic and multicultural metropolis in the United States.

I really liked my new subspecialty — forensic pathology. I had been working in the field of pathology for about nineteen years. In the Soviet Union and Israel I worked as a pathologist in hospitals, which was a great help in my present job. Forensic pathology was a mixture of many elements that made it fascinating and never boring. In spite of my years of experience, I had to solve a lot of puzzles requiring skills from various branches of medicine, as well as the approach of a forensic investigator and just common sense. Most of our cases were cases of natural death at home. We needed family and prior medical information, but we often did not have it and had to base our diagnosis solely on our findings. Homicides, accidents, suicides, sudden death of children, and all kinds of other suspicious cases required investigation by a medical examiner. We worked closely with police and often got valuable information from them. We had an excellent group of specially trained medical investigators who provided us with evidence from the scene of the death, information from the hospitals, and highly valuable details on cases of sudden infant death and when child abuse was suspected in cases of child death. We worked on a lot of public cases that TV and newspapers described rightly and wrongly. Any mistakes we made could easily become very public and humiliating to us. During my lengthy career as a medical examiner I have had a lot of public cases and other professionally challenging cases that I would like to talk about. I have presented some selected cases in my lecture "Challenging Cases in Forensic Pathology" that I periodically gave as an assistant professor at NYU for residents, fellows, and students.

We dealt a lot with hospital cases. Strictly speaking, we had to autopsy only the cases involving therapeutic complications. But in reality we were doing many more than those, because as soon as the hospital doctors see a "request" for an autopsy from the family, they refer those cases to us. Very often families like us to perform the autopsy when a patient dies in the hospital, because they consider us to be impartial. And they are right; we are independent from the hospitals. We work with the hospital doctors to find necessary information, going over the medical charts when necessary. We systematically talk with families often distressed by the death of their loved one. And of course, we often work with the lawyers, mainly prosecutors and defense attorneys, but sometimes also with lawyers in civil cases. We also participated in teaching students, fellows, and visiting doctors. The variety of activity kept me alert and organized. I, like other forensic pathologists, developed certain routines in dealing with cases because the details of every case might become legal evidence and had to be supervised responsibly. Cases can come back and surprise you, as my experience taught me.

***

Working in this office from 1986 I was involved more than once in cases in which there were multiple fatalities, such as the fire in the Bronx nightclub, many plane crashes, and of course the September 11 World Trade Center disaster.

One day in the spring of 1990 I came into the Manhattan office earlier than usual, without listening to the morning news, and was very surprised by the presence of the chief and other important people in the management of emergency events. "Something serious must have happened." And it was so: Many young people without obvious traumatic injuries were lying dead in the basement of our office. They were victims of carbon monoxide poisoning from a fire in a nightclub. This was my first encounter with a multiple-casualty disaster. In Detroit I had participated in training for handling a plane crash, but this was a real disaster. I was amazed at the efficiency shown by my boss, and David Schomburg, and a few others in organizing our work. There were no panic, no unnecessary actions; everything was to the point. As the doctor on duty that day, I was supposed to triage the cases, but I was very glad when the chief took over for me. At the end of the long day, working hard and being tired, I accidentally stuck a needle in my finger. By the next morning my finger and part of my hand had become red and swollen, despite having started a course of antibiotics the same evening, after visiting the emergency department at neighboring Bellevue Hospital. I needed more than that. I had to spend a week in Cabrini Hospital, where I was given intravenous antibiotics and surgical manipulation to prevent severe lymphangitis.

In May of 2002, for the first time since I had begun working in this office, Mayor Bloomberg invited our doctors to breakfast in Gracie Mansion. It was a sign of appreciation for our work and it was especially nice because not one of the three previous mayors, Koch, Dinkins, and Giuliani had ever invited us. The picture of Mayor Bloomberg shaking my hand that now hangs in my living room elevates my image in the eyes of my children and grandchildren. They did not pay much attention to my modest explanation that to have this picture taken we stood on a line, and the photo opportunity was repeated for every participating doctor. But I was still very proud that the mayor of the greatest City in America had received me. I had a similar experience two years later, when our office was again invited to Gracie Mansion along with a few others from the Health Department. The line for meeting the mayor was longer this time. In the new picture the mayor looked much thinner (diet or a lot of stress?) and I looked happier because of his words "Nice to see you again." Did he really remember me? Or was it the "gesture of a politician," as our toxicology chief told me (but did he say the same to her?).

As a medical examiner I often had to testify in courts. In spite of my significant experience in that, I was always excited and even a little nervous about preparing for a court appearance. Doing so was a part of the work of a medical examiner, and people's fates were involved. I had first testified in court back in Michigan during my fellowship. I learned from the beginning that criminal lawyers had to be familiar with forensic stuff in order to understand and ask the right questions. Dr. Spitz even used to give a training course for Michigan lawyers. He recommended that they study his and Dr. Fisher's book *Medicolegal Investigation of Death*, which was written in simple, understandable language for laypeople, definitely helpful to the smart lawyers. When I mentioned to Dr. Spitz that they, the lawyers, might learn our professional secrets, Dr. Spitz answered that it would be good and easier for us to deal with prepared and educated lawyers. That was an excellent reply. I was surprised by how little the criminal lawyers in New York, particularly the public defenders, knew about forensic pathology. Following Dr. Spitz's advice, I always tried to discuss the case with the lawyers before the trial, showing them our books with photos and the chapters relevant to the case; and this proved useful for all the lawyers. Some of the questions asked by the public defense lawyers during my court testimonies showed that they did not always do their homework. Perhaps they did not understand that our mission was to be objective witnesses. Of course on other occasions, I saw smart and excellently prepared prosecutors or defense lawyers, and it was a pleasure to deal with them.

One day I testified in a Manhattan court in the case of a jeweler who had been viciously killed by two men in a Manhattan store. I was sitting in the full courtroom waiting for the trial to begin. People seated on the right side of the room were speaking Russian and people on the left side were speaking Hebrew; one of the alleged killers was of Russian origin, the other Israeli. I was sitting there, and no one knew me or noticed me. I understood the conversations from both sides, thinking that very soon my testimony would start and all these people, relatives and acquaintances of the defendants, would learn of my Russian and Israeli history. Both defendants were young men in their late twenties and had translators in addition to their lawyers. The Russian defendant had one of the best defense lawyers in New York. The lawyer immediately noticed me when he came in, giving me a friendly smile and even acknowledging that this was my last working day before going on vacation. I was afraid that he might spoil my vacation by extending my testimony into the next day by asking too many questions, which defense lawyers sometimes did. But to my surprise, he did not ask me any questions, focusing instead on other parts of the prosecutor's presentation. That was smart, because what I had already described was graphic enough and disturbing for the jury, and he did not want his questions to prolong the description of the terrible injuries. I never learned the result of this trial, as I don't always know the results of trials in which I participated. But thinking about this particular trial I identified with the immigrant Russian and Israeli families who were present. We all came to this country to survive and succeed, but some of them had definitely lost this opportunity. By the way, one of our forensic pathologists, also an immigrant from the Soviet Union, was afraid to testify in another trial in which the defendant was a Russian, because of the threat of vengeance. I never worried about that possibility because we had no knowledge of who had committed the crime we testified about. We simply presented medical evidence about the cause of death and manner of death based on our objective investigation.

Over the years I discovered the strange fact that the close relatives of victims often want to hear our testimony despite the often disturbing and graphic description of severe injuries to their loved ones. I do not have an explanation for this phenomenon. I think that I myself would not like to hear all that because the picture of the suffering would be forever in front of me.

SEPTEMBER 11

It was a usual day, early morning, and I was in the autopsy room of the Bronx Medical Examiner's office when somebody came in and asked me to come to our detectives' room. There I saw repeatedly on the TV screen the scene of an airplane crashing into the North Tower of the World Trade Center. "My God!" I exclaimed, "this is a terrorist attack." "No," one of our detectives said, "it's a commuter plane accident." Unfortunately I was right, and the next thing we saw, now in real time, was another airplane crashing into the South Tower. Shocked, we were glued to the TV, and then the unbelievable happened in front of our terrified eyes — both buildings collapsed like a house of cards! I was sure that the same question was on everybody's mind: "How many people were killed there, ten or twenty thousand?" We did not even have the words or even dare to say that. I called Sam, who fortunately just a half a year ago had moved to a midtown location from the fifty-seventh floor of the South Tower. He had proudly had a corner office there, and on a good day all Manhattan was "under his feet." Sam was overwhelmed with emotion and could not say a single word. I knew that our older son Leonid was farther away from this area, and Sam eventually told me on the telephone that our younger son, very worried, had called Sam's cell from Massachusetts, fearing that his father might still be in the Tower. I also called my friend Nadia Savitsky whose husband Victor worked in the World Financial Center. She told me that he was already at home alive and unhurt, that he had gone right away to the garage where his car was parked, and without stopping, he had driven home to Queens.

The events of September 11 amounted to a huge disaster and a huge calamity. The Office of the Medical Examiner quickly became ready to do whatever was necessary. All four of our doctors from the Bronx were sent to Manhattan. I was left in the Bronx office to cover our everyday load alone because we could not interrupt our routine service. Dr. J. was on vacation somewhere at sea on a sailboat. She was expected back in a few days to join me working in the Bronx. Our main office switched to the twenty-four-hour doctors' schedule, expecting to meet a workload caused by thousands of bodies. But the unusually high temperature at the disaster site caused evaporation or disintegration of the bodies, and we were receiving thousands of bones instead of whole bodies. I do not think that any office in the world had ever had to handle such an unbelievably gruesome, difficult task as identifying the victims during the many months that followed. Behind the bodies, small and large bones, fragments of civilian clothing and of firefighters and police uniforms, documents and pictures, were people who were gone and people who left with broken lives, disrupted families, disrupted financial status, multiple unanswered questions such as "Why?" or "Is this true?" or "Are you sure that he or she was there?" or "How can this be?"

The symbol of New York City, the Twin Towers, had disappeared. The disaster was so huge and unreal that it was difficult to comprehend. The strong smell of a burned house became a lasting feature of our beautiful city for months to come. The gray smoke in the sky stayed for many days. The same day the Towers fell I went for a walk in my neighborhood and saw people in the stores going about their everyday business, or having coffee and eating something. There was no panic on their faces; nobody was buying more than usual for fear of food shortages. I immediately recalled my life experience in Israel and my amazement there at the continuation of normal life despite the terrorist attacks and frequent disasters. I also was a child of WWII, with all the consequences during and after that war in Russia and Ukraine. Even with all those experiences, I still had a hard time comprehending these events and the evidence of normal life that accompanied them. I saw evidence of a new spirit of unity. American flags were everywhere, and not for a day or two but for months to come. In the next few days we visited the small neighboring firehouse to pay tribute and donate money on behalf of the families of the eight firefighters they lost in one day. The pictures, the flowers, the grief . . . All looked so surrealistic, yet it was our reality.

Our office became very focused, well organized, no complaints, no panic. Everybody knew what we were supposed to do, as if we had experienced it before. A team of doctors and police officers was on duty in the Manhattan office 24/7. A support team of radiologists, photographers, dentists, and a forensic anthropologist was always on duty as well. The team of medical investigators and police officers together with the computer support personnel were gathering and analyzing all materials for identification of victims in the auditorium where we usually held our weekly conferences. That was the most important part of our job. The cause of death was clear, but most bodies were absent. Our office was faced with the gigantic task of handling and preserving the unusual material that was brought to us instead of the bodies. The office also handled the great many telephone calls from the desperate families. The serology lab under Dr. Shaler played an outstanding role in the identification process because we had to deal with so many disparate small fragments of bones instead of whole bodies. Recently evolved DNA tests became a primary tool for this unprecedented by scope investigation. A lot of legal issues had to be dealt with. Nobody had any experience like this before. During my fifteen years of work in this office we "only" handled a couple of airplane disasters and the Bronx nightclub fire, which left ninety young people dead, all from high carbon monoxide levels and burns. But this was very different in scale and evidence. I knew for sure that our boss, Dr. Hirsch, and his direct subordinates, like David Schomburg or Dr. Shaler, had never had any experience like this before.

I could not forget the repeated rituals of the firefighters and police officers when they brought in the remains of their own colleagues. They would arrange themselves in double file and greet everybody with a salute and pain on their faces, and I was sure that they thought in this moment, as all of us did, that these bodies could otherwise have been their own. And this encounter was repeated over and over again. Our work was always connected to the work of the police, and we relied on evidence they provided to us. We worked with police officers during the routine identification in homicide cases. We also often met them in the courts when they testified, as we did. But now I and my colleagues experienced a special feeling of solidarity and closeness. In turn, we saw from the police officers and all others great respect for everything that we were doing. We spent hours and hours together. I was very glad to find out that one of our unmarried doctors met her future husband there, a handsome police officer with dark hair and absolutely stunning blue eyes. After nine months they had a daughter and after another year they had a son. Such circumstances increase people's appreciation for life, families, and friends. The medical career alone no longer seemed of primary importance.

Six months after the event, our doctors were invited for breakfast with Mayor Bloomberg at Gracie Mansion as a sign of his appreciation for our work. We heard many good words about our office and its role in facing the challenges of September 11. In the following years lectures have been given at universities and to various professional societies considering the massive disaster and the unprecedented work of the OCME.

Sam took the September 11 events very personally. After all, he had spent the previous eleven years in a Wall Street industry, mostly revolving around its downtown offices. Not long before, Sam had left Bridge Information Systems (located on the 57th–

58th floors of the South Tower) for an executive position with a hedge fund, and he took with him a group of programmers with whom he worked closely. Two of them, Dino and Natalya, approached Sam on September 10 to sign a voucher for their registration for a professional conference to be held the next day on the 110th floor of the North Tower, at Windows on the World. After some hesitation, Sam, who usually signed everything for his favorite employees, refused this time, saying that the voucher was quite expensive, considering for the not-so-good business outlook. Well, nobody returned from that conference. The next morning Sam received a call from London from the organizers of the conference asking the whereabouts of the two registrants, Dino and Natalya. Sam thanked God for keeping them alive! Both friends framed Sam's e-mail and hung the copies in their offices. Another of Sam's colleagues from his previous job, Weibin W., left Sam's firm for Cantor Fitzgerald. He disappeared with all of them. We have at home a present he once gave us — a pen-and-pencil holder made from a curved horn.

MY RECENT YEARS

I continued working as a medical examiner in the Office of the Chief Medical Examiner, where I was one of the few doctors who had been there for so long. I have survived the three chiefs and three direct deputies. Some of our doctors have successfully relocated, becoming chief medical examiners in other states, in part because our office is one of the most experienced and respected. Some other doctors during those years relocated not so successfully, quit, or just disappeared from view. I find it strange that very few retain connections with us after they move on. Probably it is natural or really "American" not to be sentimental and nostalgic.

Almost all the foreign-origin doctors no longer worked here, except for a few from Haiti in the Brooklyn office. Now we employed mostly American graduates, some of them from the best medical schools. The long list of applicants for our forensic fellowship program was a source of pride for our management. Even residents of pathology from Yale Medical School started systematically to appear in our Bronx office every two weeks (thanks to our deputy, the graduate of the same pathology residency at Yale) and we, the attending physicians, were teaching them. Nothing new — for years I have been teaching the students from NYU in my role as an assistant professor in the Forensic Pathology Department.

In the Bronx I was the last of the Mohicans of the old timers — all the other doctors were younger. I liked to work with them and really did not feel my age. And in fact my life and professional experience gave me confidence and provided a basis for the positive attitude of my colleagues toward me. I personally liked to share and show what I was doing and listened to different opinions and, to be honest, I was not afraid to disagree with my boss. My fearlessness caused me some trouble in the not-so-long past but I survived. I liked our weekly conferences; they provided a forum for new thoughts and created in me a good feeling that I was at the front edge of my profession. The deputy, with whom I have worked for the last few years, was in his late thirties, intelligent, knowledgeable, and a very decent colleague, and I think that he could become the chief of the office when our current boss retires.

In recent years our field of medicine has become very popular on TV and in the press, partially because of our work on the September 11 disaster and also because of the many court shows about highly publicized criminal cases and the gruesome details of the autopsy reports. This really surprises me. I do not like the relatively young "former" prosecutors and defense lawyers, probably highly paid, who participate on the Larry King show, discussing — often very incompetently — forensic pathology issues. Why are all of them "former" so early? I do like though the TV show with the "former" Judge "Judy." It is fun to watch her. She definitely knows what she is talking about, and she applies her real courtroom experience as well as common sense. I never dealt with her in the New York courts but I know her husband, a smart Bronx judge with whom I dealt in many cases, including one very public case of death in police custody. I also saw him once as a "former" prosecutor and the current TV court judge, but he is definitely not as successful as his wife in this role; she exhibits a great sense of humor despite her long career in the courts.

"I love stories and my writing is principally concentrated on stories, but not with a pretense of scientific precision" – Mario Vargas Llosa, Peruvian novelist

PART 2
SELECTED STORIES

MUMMY

It was one of those unusual days which happens every four years—February 29, and it still was very early in the morning, so I decided against driving but rather walked from my East 79th street to our office at East 30th Street in lower Manhattan. It took me some forty-five minutes of really brisk walking. The morning was lovely, crisp, and cool. As always, New York was busy and beautiful at this time of the day. People were carrying that particular "New Yorkish" chic that you would not find in other cities.

For one thing, you could not miss those unique, yet typical for New York, dog-walkers. It was amazing how they handled in one bundle so many dogs of different breeds, ages, and behaviors. And those stuck-together, numerous dogs would not fight, but rather walk simultaneously and proudly, each maintaining its individual frequency of steps, according to leg length, and managing to keep the same speed.

I personally was not able to properly train our only dog, the red Doberman-pincher Gingi, loved by my entire family. As a result of my "training," every morning and evening all the doormen of our neighborhood smiled widely and watched me, a small and delicately-built woman running behind a sixty-five pound muscular dog on a leash. "Who is walking whom?" they tirelessly asked me. I was not always in a mood to answer them.

After my forty-five minute walk, I came to the office. The simple truth about our office—it was never boring. Almost every day we were getting some "excitement"—either too many cases, a high profile case (like police shooting, police brutality, or child abuse), or even an air-crash disaster or a fire with multiple victims, and so on and so on. I think that because of the constant excitement, I was all the time on the move, even on my vacations. I could not simply rest on a beach enjoying the sun and sounds of the ocean like most people did. I would always walk miles along the beach until I was almost completely exhausted.

Today was no different; we were very busy: four autopsies and four external examinations for me alone. Among the other cases, I noticed a strange one—a seventy year old black female who had been found in the bedroom of a private house. Her body had been mummified! And the family was living in the same house! The case had already made a furor, and many people from different labs were coming to look at the mummy. The body was entirely mummified, indeed. It really was an unusual-looking body; it had the appearance of an Egyptian mummy from the Metropolitan Museum! I did not expect that in this day and age we had the knowledge of how to preserve a dead body in such a manner.

The body was that of a well-developed black female, appearing to be consistent with the stated age of seventy years, measuring five feet, five inches, and weighing only seventy pounds. Our chief technician helped me open that brown, stone-like body with a saw. The head hair was absent except for the braids on both sides. These braids were covered by whitish salt crystals. The same material was present everywhere on the body, covering stony-looking wrinkles of the skin. The soft tissue was completely absent on the face. The tongue also had the consistency of dark brown stone. There were no signs of trauma on the head, or any other part of the body, for that matter.

The internal examination revealed a moderate degree of atherosclerosis. All organs showed autolysis but were in a very good recognizable state. The heart was small, weighing only eighty grams (normally it should be around two hundred and fifty grams). Both lungs were collapsed, and the right lung weighed one hundred and fifty grams, the left, eighty grams (normally each would be three to four hundred grams). The stomach was empty.

Upon completion of the autopsy, I made the case "pending further study," meaning that conclusions required an examination by a toxicology lab as well as the results of the police investigation. I did a lot of photography. For histology and toxicology, I sent small pieces of the internal organs—brain, liver and kidney—and also the white salt-like material from the skin. And of course, an x-ray was done prior to my starting the autopsy.

The story I received from the smart and diligent police detective was very unusual, even for a sophisticated New Yorker and a "nothing could surprise me" medical examiner. The deceased had lived with her daughter, son-in-law, and grandson in a private house. Her sister, who lived in Florida, had not heard from her for two years. She started to worry and called the police, asking them to check on the well-being of her sister. A few months prior, the NYPD had done as requested, but without actually seeing the old lady, and had accepted the daughter's information that everything was fine. Yet, the lady from Florida had not been satisfied because such a long silence was unusual for her sister. In addition, her relationship with the niece was not so good, and she felt that the niece could not be trusted.

"My sister has diabetes, and I suspect something may have happened," she said when she called the police again to request a new investigation.

This time the detective insisted on seeing the old lady. The daughter did not refuse and brought him to her mother's room. The room measured approximately fourteen by fourteen feet and was in a very neat condition. A bureau on the right side of the bed had a Bible and a crucifix on it. A stand with rubber gloves and diaper pads on the surface was on the left side. A blowing fan was positioned at the center of the room. The mummified body of the old lady was lying face up on the bed with a hospital type diaper in place. Another diaper pad covered the body from the neck to the thigh.

After recovering from the initial shock, the detective asked, "How long has this woman been dead?"

"She is not dead," answered the daughter. "She is in a different stage of her life, in a stage of animation."

The daughter also explained to the police investigator that she had a very special love for her mother and that her mother "was not the way she appeared to be now." The daughter had a number of nursing degrees and was a superior at one of the nursing schools. She said,

"I probably have more degrees than your medical examiners and knowledge of things they do not have."

The daughter's husband and her teenager son did not dare to enter the room during this period of one and a half years and did not realize the condition of the old lady. They were satisfied with the explanation: "Don't worry, she is fine. I am taking care of her."

And she did take care of her mother, diligently and scrupulously preserving her body as a mummy. Both the husband and the son also insisted that the house did not have any odor and in no way differed from before. The case looked very strange, to say at least, and the mummy was taken to the Office of Medical Examiner. The daughter, in turn, was examined by a psychiatrist who diagnosed her as having some kind of a borderline disorder, but she was not considered a threat for society.

An x-ray of the body did not reveal anything unusual. The toxicological study was also negative. Our anthropologist studied the case and gave the detailed description with a conclusion. It was not unusual to see mummified remains among forensic anthropological cases in New York. Mummified tissue occurs naturally under hot/dry or cold/dry conditions. Natural mummification in New York City generally takes anywhere from one to three years or more. The body of the old lady presented strikingly unusual features in contrast to natural mummification.

There was no doubt at all that the body was mummified, but the degree of mummification was inconsistent with natural processes, as observed in other cases. In this instance, the external tissue (skin) was absolutely rock hard (not at all pliable) and bright orange in color, while the internal preservation was quite moist. This is clearly indicative of artificial, intentional mummification as practiced by some cultures in the distant past. The application of olive oil in combination with a dry enclosed space (such as her bedroom) would accomplish this state of mummification quite rapidly over time. The white powder found all over the body was identified as small salt crystals.

Base on the autopsy and all the other information, I put in the certificate the cause of death as "Atherosclerotic cardiovascular disease. Diabetes mellitus. Manner: natural."

This case reminded me *Psycho*, the classic movie by Alfred Hitchcock, with Anthony Perkins in the role of Norman Bates, the multiple-personality owner of the "Bates Motel," who mummified his mother. To be honest, I do not believe in multiple personalities. One is the real, and others are for cover-up, but this is beside the point. Let us leave it for psychiatrists. Fortunately, nobody was killed in this case.

EXOTIC DANCER

A thirty-four year old Hispanic woman was found in her apartment by police after a call made because of the odor arising from the tenth floor apartment in the Bronx. The neighbors, an elderly couple from the Dominican Republic, had not seen her recently, but they did pay attention to a note attached to the door. It was dated May 24, was in the super's calligraphic writing, and concerned an overdue rent payment.

The young woman had moved into this apartment recently and was seen rarely, mostly at odd hours. These neighbors did not really know much about her except that "she was quiet, kept to herself, and had some kind of night job, coming home early mornings." Nobody visited her, and she would not talk, but acknowledged others with slight nod and a mild tired smile of recognition when she happened to run onto a neighbor at such early hour.

"She was so beautiful and a little mysterious with her straight shiny dark long hair, deep-seated, slightly oval eyes, and slim, gracious body," said the tall, gray-haired neighbor. He was accompanied by his small and slightly plump wife whose eyes were full of tears. "So young and beautiful, and already dead," she added.

The door of the apartment was locked and had to be opened by force by the police. All the windows were locked shut. The apartment was "lived in and orderly," a detective wrote in his report. The report mentioned "a crack pipe with alleged crack still in the pipe" as well as "alleged crack in a white container" that were found there. Drug paraphernalia and two empty pill containers were also found, along with several loose pills on the bed. The poor young woman was discovered face-up on the bedroom floor of her one-bedroom apartment. She might have been in this position for two to three weeks, considering the decomposition of the body and the insects present in the apartment. She was dressed in dark pants and white socks without anything else. Her long hair and her face were covered by maggots. Detectives also discovered a computer, a cellular phone with her last call dated two weeks earlier, a safe with a large amount of jewelry, a wallet, and an identification card. The safe was opened by the detectives, and a total of $24,000 was discovered in possession of the deceased. A lot of pictures depicting this woman as an exotic dancer were found in the safe. She had been photographed while performing belle and striptease dances. Her long straight hair surrounded the delicate Indian-type face with sad deep brown eyes and slightly protuberant lips. In the photos, the long, thin body of the dancer exhibited small and beautifully shaped breasts and a narrow waist smoothly widening into proportionally built hips with the barely-covered triangle.

It was in our Bronx Office where I performed the autopsy. Nothing unusual was discovered. An x-ray was done to exclude gunshot wounds or other trauma and for the purposes of identification because the body was unrecognizable. We could not show it to relatives or acquaintances when they came for identification. Photography, as always, was done for documentation. Small samples of blood, bile, brain, and liver tissue were taken for toxicology. The woman had breast implants, and that by itself could also help with the identification, in addition to the usual means such as scars, birth marks, x-rays of the body, dental x-rays, and fingerprints. Usually, it remains in our judgment which of the above is necessary in each case. After the autopsy, my diagnosis was "pending further study." I was waiting for the toxicology report.

In addition to the police report, usually called a DD5, I also received a few pages with a mug shot pedigree (I did not know at first, what that meant). It was a picture of the same woman, though not looking too happy, with her name, physical description, and the description of the cause for her arrest the previous summer for criminal possession of stolen property. Whoa!

From the cellular phone of the deceased, the detectives found the name of a young man whom they approached. He introduced himself as her boyfriend. It turned out that the young man had already been to the police twice to file reports about her disappearance two weeks earlier. Just recently, he had been approached by her family, which he was not aware of before, regarding her whereabouts.

The young man—white, with a Scandinavian last name—was in his middle thirties and worked successfully in the Wall Street industry. He spent his free time on golf courses, and in nightclubs, where he was introduced to this astonishingly beautiful young woman. She started living with him. But the strange thing was that he knew very little about his beautiful girlfriend, who managed to keep him in the dark concerning her secret life, her night work, and even her rental apartment in the Bronx. Very often, she would leave for "tax accounting work" in some Hoboken firm that at least twice a week required her to work a night shift. Busy with his demanding Wall Street life, he did not mind. He did not worry about her until she did not show up and did not return his calls to her cell phone. This was especially unusual because they were planning, after her yoga class and his golf, to spend the evening and the night together. He had tried calling the firm where she supposedly worked, but the agency was not listed in Hoboken.

The Wall Street man was in shock upon receiving the bad news from the police. He denied any knowledge about his girlfriend's drug activity. He provided police with the phone numbers of the deceased's uncle and cousin, whom I contacted shortly after the autopsy. The cousin and uncle did not know much about the girl, her apartment, her drug usage, or even her professional activity.

The cousin told me that the mother of the deceased lived in the Dominican Republic. I asked the cousin if the deceased had had any surgery. "Only breast implants," was her answer. That helped with the identification, especially since we did not have either her doctor's name, if any, or her dentist and dental x-rays. And of course, her previous summer arrest helped with her fingerprint identification.

In a few weeks, as expected, I received the toxicology report. It revealed that the deceased had in her blood a small amount of ethanol, which might result from decomposition, plus small amounts of cocaine and its metabolites benzoylecgonine, opiates, and nordizepam. I concluded that the cause of death was acute intoxication caused by all these combined drugs and medication.

***

In my teenage years, the time with no TV, iPod music, computer games, or SMS messaging, when I mostly busied myself with non-stop reading, I read *Notes of the Psychiatrist* by Lydia Bogdanovich and *Notes of the Physician* by Veresaev. Of course, I also read a lot of stories by Chekhov, the great writer and physician. And perhaps because I wanted to become a physician for as long as I can remember, I clearly remember these books where medical cases were described in their complicity, curiosity, and simply humanity. The authors, by combining their skills as medical doctors and writers, made these everyday cases into vivid and interesting stories, delving deeply in the causes, circumstances, and consequences of the cases.

Forensic pathologists deal with the most tragic, sad, unexpected, strange, and sometimes unexplained ends of human life. We do not know these people. We see only their dead bodies and try to find the causes of their deaths, and then patiently and sensitively explain the findings to their loved ones. Our conclusions are based on the circumstances surrounding the deaths, on police reports, and on autopsy findings augmented with everything available from modern test technology. We talk with relatives before and after an autopsy and tactfully ask some questions which might shed light on the cause of death. We talk with the hospital and with clinic doctors to find necessary medical information from when the deceased was alive. But we still do not know a lot of things about these people because we never knew them and never talked to them.

That is why, in the case of the exotic dancer, I could only ask but could not answer such questions as:

- How could this young and beautiful lady have ended up drugged, dead, decomposed, and alone?

- How could the young and successful man have been so out of touch with his girlfriend as not to discover her double life?

- Was he clean of drugs?

- Why did he never call me about the final result?

PRINCE AND PRINCESS

It is an April evening in early nineties. The evening news makes a sensational pronouncement: a royal couple has been found dead in their off-Park-Avenue condominium. According to the news, it was a murder-suicide. My husband Sam and I go for our routine one-hour evening walk, and I head toward the street of the crime, only several blocks southwest from our co-op building. The TV people with their equipment are still there, but there is no crowd. The elegant brownstone building looks peaceful and rich, with lights in the windows of both lower floors. Only the third floor windows are dark. "It must have happened there," I think while walking with Sam along the street. There is not much action. Nobody is coming in or out of the building; the street is empty and quiet. We continue our walk, pretending that we do not know and do not see anything. Tomorrow I will be in charge of the autopsies and will take the case for myself. I do not know yet into what I will be putting myself!

The next morning, as expected, I am placed in charge of these two cases. The initial information is that the husband, a fifty-seven year old West Indian man, has been stabbed in the neck by his jealous wife. But it is not clear why his wife, a seventy-two year old white woman, is dead. Has she committed a suicide, taking some pills that were found in the apartment by the investigators of the scene? They both were heard on Friday afternoon having a very loud family dispute, so loud that the maid had left early to avoid the scene. The same maid found them both dead on Monday morning, and she called the police. Initial investigation by the police gives me information that this is a case of homicide-suicide.

I proceed to the morgue where I observe the bodies of the husband with his stab wound to the neck and of the wife, and the latter looks more decomposed than her husband. "I will do the husband first," is my decision.

The man is fully clad in a black jacket, a white shirt with a black-reddish tie, dark gray trousers, black shoes, and blue socks. Strangely, he does not have underwear. He is a well-developed, good-looking man (in spite of some decomposition). He is five feet, nine inches in height, and he weighs one hundred and sixty-five pounds. He has thick dark-brown hair and brown slightly bulging eyes. The face has dark-bluish discoloration with multiple reddish abrasions of the protuberant areas. The same areas have slippage of the skin. The conjunctives (the mucous membranes that line the inner surface of the eyelids) have conglomerated areas of bleeding ("hemorrhage" is the word of Latin origin that medical doctors use). These hemorrhages of the eyes and the face are like a red light for us. I think about asphyxia (suffocation). There could be many causes of asphyxia. On the other hand, these bleedings on the mucosal surface of the eyes might simply appear on a body found in a face down position, as this man was. They also could be a result of resuscitation efforts; however, this man had none. The slippage of skin that I noticed on the face, chest, left knee, and both elbows is a sign of decomposition that usually appears forty-eight hours after death, depending on the temperature, the condition of the body, the presence of clothes on the body, and other factors. Mild mummification of the man's hands is also present. Mummification is the shrinkage of the skin that takes place as a body dries in the first few days after death, if it is located in a dry atmosphere. On my external examination, I see a one and a quarter inch long horizontal cut on the neck, followed on the left side with a one and a half inch superficial horizontal abrasion.

I proceed to the internal examination. I find a big and very important surprise! The neck wound turns out to be a very superficial cut that does not penetrate or perforate any organ or blood vessel of the neck. This wound could not have killed the man. The autopsy shows soft tissue bleeding of both sides of the head. This might be a result of decomposition, but it also might be the result of a blunt force injury to the head.

I call my boss, the chief of the Office of Medical Examiners, and I show him my findings. We do not jump to any conclusions yet.

I start to perform the autopsy of the man's wife. She is a petite woman, five feet, three inches tall and one hundred and forty-five pounds. Her decomposition is much more pronounced than of her husband. This is especially obvious on the face, neck, and upper chest. There is slippage of skin on different areas of the body. There is also marbling of the skin due to hemolysis of blood in superficial vessels. On the right hand, below the small finger, I find a stab wound, a half-inch long and a half-inch in depth. The woman has dark red manicure with well-shaped, cleaned, and polished nails, which looks strange on this broken, greenish, lifeless body. The autopsy shows an enlarged heart and signs of atherosclerosis. She has atherosclerotic and hypertensive cardiovascular disease, usual findings for her age. If she had been found under different circumstances, we would have suspected nothing unusual. But the two bodies in the same apartment are definitely unusual and very suspicious!

After the autopsy, I call the detective and tell him that my findings are more consistent with double homicide by suffocation. It does not match their initial homicide-suicide theory, so I request a more thorough investigation. For the time being, I put the cause of death as "pending further study," and the manner, CUPPI (circumstances unclear, pending police investigation). I rush these cases for the toxicology and microscopic studies of organs, and I wait for the more detailed police investigation.

The medical investigator, who was initially on the scene, brings me a small but very important bit of information—a little piece of dark duct tape has been noticed in the deceased man's hair and was vouched by the police. Why was it there? The detective does not offer any explanation. And another detail—two bloodied cotton balls were found near the woman's body in the bedroom.

The couple was last seen alive at approximately 4:00 PM on Friday and was discovered by their maid at 10:22 AM on Monday. Their building has twenty-four hour doorman service and is equipped with six-screen surveillance cameras, so the police detectives must study this information. According to the medical investigator's report, the apartment appeared to be ransacked with some papers scattered on the floor. Also, the report indicates presence of blood in different areas of the apartment. The same medical investigator (not a police detective) also tells me that there was a small piece of duct tape on the man's tie.

My boss comes up with the suggestion that we visit the apartment ourselves, and we do. The police detectives join us. The couple lived in a European-style decorated apartment in the Manhattan's Upper-East brownstone. In the living room, on the wooden floor with no carpet, we see a brushing blood stain. The living room is connected through the hall with the bedroom and a bathroom on the right. There are blood spots in the living room leading to the hall and then to the bathroom. In the bathroom, there is a soft tissue box that probably was used by the woman trying to stop the bleeding from her finger cut. Her husband's body was found face-down on the floor of the living room, and she, face-up on the floor of their bedroom. In the hall connecting the living room, bathroom, and the bedroom, the police had discovered a piece of paper with a hesitating woman's writing, "Chase." Why did she write that? The telephone cord was disconnected in the kitchen and in the living room. Everything we have observed so far is not that innocent; on the contrary, it looks extremely suspicious: the brushing bloody stains on the living room floor are consistent with violent movement of the head and the autopsy finding of the soft tissue bleeding of the head. The blood spots in the hall and bathroom are from the finger wound of the dead woman. So far, the police information that the wife stabbed her husband and then committed suicide by taking some pills does not substantiate.

According to the building doorman, two men visited the couple on the Friday after the housekeeper left. The couple apparently knew these men because they allowed them into the apartment. The two men, who were unknown to the doorman, had left the couple's apartment after a while with a small package. The doorman had heard the man's voice from upstairs saying good-bye to the guests. According to the police, nothing disappeared from the apartment.

The local newspapers were full of rumors and other information. The couple was known in high society as the Prince and Princess. According to the New York newspapers, the Prince had a reputation as an independently wealthy man who invested in a wide variety of businesses. His ancestors were famous maharajas. A few years earlier, he had announced that he was investing in a joint venture with clothing designer, Gene Meyer, and a Japanese firm, but later the deal fell through when he did not provide the millions in financing required to launch the line. The Princess had been born in Brazil, and she had been a wealthy widow when she married him ten years ago. Her style was more subdued. She was less flamboyant than her husband. She was more cultured and laid back. Among the charities supported by the couple were the National Symphony Orchestra and the American Society for Preservation of Russian Culture. They played bridge. He loved women.

As I contemplated these cases during the next sleepless night, I imagined the following scenario: The two men who came to the Prince and Princess's apartment demanded something (such as money or jewelry). They covered the victims' mouths with a duct tape. This is why the neighbors did not hear the couple, who usually were very loud. The woman, scared to death with the tape on her mouth, wrote on the piece of paper the name of the bank where they kept their money, and probably their jewelry, as well. The assailants also demanded something from the Prince, putting the ligature over his neck, applying pressure, restricting his breathing, and striking his head violently against the wooden floor. The Prince lost consciousness and then his life. The something that pressed his neck was quickly taken off, and that was why the ligature mark was very faint. The woman could be easily smothered by anything like a pillow or a blanket. But how the doorman could hear the "good-bye" from the Prince to these men? Was he wrong, mislead, or also involved in this matter?

The next morning, I go my boss's office very early. He is fresh and energetic from his routine workout at the health club. Very excited, I rush to explain my vision and scenario. Despite my excitement, I notice the boss's wet T-shirt on the hanger in the open closet and appreciate his dedication to the health. He listens to me attentively but without my excitement. He is "cool," as always, but he is definitely not in disagreement with me. We wait for the lab.

The toxicology report excludes any drug overdose or abuse, and the microscopic study of internal organs does not reveal anything except the atherosclerotic changes of internal organs expected for a seventy-two year old lady. Careful study of the Kodachromes shows the one-inch-wide, whitish ligature mark on the man's neck even more pronounced than at autopsy. This and the bleeding of the soft tissue of both sides of his head and the brushing blood spots on the floor suggest violent action in an assault. Absence of any other cause of simultaneous death of both victims leads us to the diagnosis of "homicidal asphyxia by physical means." In lay people's language, it means that they both were suffocated by strangulation, smothering, or neck compression.

But the district attorney on the case, a young smart woman in her thirties, still has her doubts and asks us to send all our findings to a well-known forensic pathologist in Miami, asking him to review the case and venture a second opinion. Soon, he writes a letter that he is in absolute agreement with our conclusions.

***

In June of the same year, we had another double homicide, this time on the West Side of Manhattan. A pianist was killed in his apartment, along with his friend, after advertising the sale of his piano in the newspaper. Both middle-aged men were killed by multiple stab-wounds. The killers were not found immediately, and nobody connected these double homicides because, at that time, the only known similarity was the double killing. Another forensic pathologist of our office performed and handled this West Side double homicide.

I did not hear anything from the detectives about my two cases until August when all of a sudden I received a call from my boss, suggesting I listen to the news on channel five. And I did. Two men were arrested in another state for a reason completely unrelated to our cases. One of them was a twenty-two year old fellow, and the other was a fifty-five year old man. The older man, after being beaten by the younger, was afraid of further hostile and irrational actions from his partner. He decided to confess to their two previous crimes in New York. The real motive for this confession turned out to be more complicated, as I learned later on.

According to the older man, they knew the Prince from the art auctions at Sotheby (such a strange acquaintance). On the day of the murders, the Prince and Princess expected to go out to dinner with these acquaintances. Both men came to their apartment, and then, according to the older man's statement, the young man started to demand something from the Prince, who strongly refused to submit. Things went wrong, and the younger man lost control and suffocated the Prince with a belt. Following his younger partner's order, the older man took the Princess to the bedroom. A little later, the younger man suffocated her with a pillow. The older man said he did not do anything except witness the crime.

The older man also confessed to another crime—the June double homicide on the West Side. The composer and his friend were viciously stabbed at the composer's apartment because the robbery did not go well. The older man expressed his fear of his partner who was vicious, sadistic, and unpredictable. He said he did not kill anybody, but was present and witnessed the murders, as he had in the case of the Prince and Princess killings.

The two suspects were brought to New York. They started accusing each other in both crimes, but as the investigation showed, they were both very serious criminals with a long trail of murders. It was not the first time the older man had confessed to a crime, but in the previous cases he had managed to escape real punishment. Fortunately, he was not that lucky this time.

The trial occurred a year later. It took place in the absolutely empty auditorium of a Manhattan courtroom. In New York, the public and the press have a very short memory indeed. The press had been very eloquent at the time of the murders and arrests. No family members of the victims or the defendants were present in the room. There were only the judge, the jury, the defense and the prosecutor, the defendants, the police officers, and me—the usual players. Each had a separate trial. In front of me, with two police officers behind him, was the first defendant, a middle-aged white man in a dark suit and a blue tie. His face, I was afraid to admit to myself, showed some attractiveness and even intelligence. He attentively watched and listened to my testimony with curiosity on his face. It was unusual because, during my testimonies, more often I have seen defendants sitting motionless without any expression. Seeing these faces, I have often thought that they must be guilty, because otherwise they would have to explode or at least show certain emotions, such as denial or disbelief. But this guy was different, very experienced and criminally shrewd. He probably thought that if his face showed big interest, his confessions would save his life again, as had happened before.

He showed agreement with what I was saying because my findings and conclusions did not contradict his story about how the crime was committed. But of course, I did not know who did what. Even though he did not look like a dangerous killer, I had to remind myself that people can be deceived by handsome killers. The Prince, for one, was deceived—he met these guys at the auction, had some kind of business relationship with them, allowed them into his residence, and had planned to dinner with them. Amazing, is it not?

I liked the district attorney on the case, a well-organized and experienced woman. She carefully and diligently prepared for the trial. She was not pushy, and she very respectfully listened to my interpretation of the autopsy findings. I liked that she let me testify without interruption, without playing small games around minor details of the findings, as some less-experienced lawyers did. I particularly liked it because I was very proud of our handling of this case from the beginning to the end.

The second defendant was absolutely different—a young man in his early twenties with smooth black hair, dark dead eyes, and a pale emotionless face. I did not see any reaction from him to anything that was showed or said in the trial. "Cold-blood killer, pathological killer, probably," I thought.

The investigation and the trial confirmed what we thought. They taped the mouth of each victim. The Prince was suffocated by a wide ligature that was then promptly taken from his neck. The Princess, at first, was with the Prince in the living room. They threaten her with a knife and stabbed her in a left-hand finger. Bleeding from the wound, she ran to the bathroom and put a paper tissue on the wound. The criminals demanded from her information about her bank account. The frightened Princess was not able to talk with her mouth taped shut, so she wrote the name of the bank with shaking hands. Then she was suffocated in her bedroom with a pillow.

Both defendants blamed each other. They both received what they deserved—twenty-five year sentences.

DISMEMBERED BODY

It is early January of 1990. I do not like this time of the year—the Holidays are over, all the festivities and parties are behind, and the mood is somber. The winter days are short. The skies are mostly gray, and snow in the city is dirty, if there is any. What is a winter without snow? So, to change my gloomy morning mood, I decide to walk some fifty-plus streets from my home at East End Avenue to our office at First and 28th. Wearing comfortable sneakers, it will take me forty-five minutes of brisk walking, about the same as taking the bus. In fifteen minutes, thanks to the adrenalin pumping from my glands, my mood starts climbing up. Eventually, in a bright mood and upbeat for work, I am entering our five-story office building, which is adjacent to New York University.

I noticed at once that it would be a busy day. Even though my two cases of drug abuse are not so difficult, my third case looks complicated and time-consuming. The night before, in the abandoned area of the Bronx, a decapitated and dismembered body had been set on fire. It was then discovered by firefighters and the police.

On the marble table, I see the dismembered body of a woman, the headless torso cut in half in the middle, the upper extremities with no hands and both legs amputated above the knees. The cut-off left leg, which was found near the body, is positioned near the torso, but the amputated right leg is absent. The body is partially burnt and covered by soot. The dark-red sweater on the upper torso, a red skirt on the lower torso, and white underwear are stained by soot and partially burnt. Our x-ray technician is making x-rays of the whole body to exclude the presence of bullets or pieces of knife—and also for identification purposes. Kenny, a photographer, is making numerous pictures of the body and clothes. I start filling up the diagram, depicting everything of importance that I see during the external examination.

The estimated weight of the deceased is around two hundred pounds, and her height is estimated at five feet, six inches to five feet, eight inches. The head and neck are absent. The neck is cut at its lower end, and the cut is sharp. The remnants of skin and soft tissue are present on the left side in the direction of three to five o'clock. The chest is symmetrical with well-developed breasts. The upper torso has a sharp horizontal cut above the diaphragm, and the inner abdominal organs protrude from this cut. The margins of the cut are dried, and there is no blood inside; therefore, the body has been cut after death of the woman. The upper torso measures fourteen inches in length. The upper extremities consist of preserved arms and forearms without hands, and the margins of the forearms are dried and obscure by fire. Two bones of the forearms are cut sharply on both sides. The left arm and forearm measures seventeen inches in length and the right, seventeen and a half inches. The lower part of torso consists of the abdomen with sharp margins, dried and obscured by soot and burns. The amputated left leg is seventeen inches long and contains the knee, lower leg, and foot. The foot is well preserved and stained by soot.

When I perform the internal examination, it does not reveal any abnormalities. The woman's heart is of normal size and weight and shows absolutely perfect aorta and coronary arteries with no atherosclerosis. This woman was a young, healthy person without any visible diseases.

So, how did she die? Was she killed, dismembered, and then set on fire to hide the crime? In that case, how was she killed? Was she shot in the absent head? Was she struck on the head with a heavy object? Was she stabbed in the neck? Or did she die by other means? She certainly did not have any capsules of cocaine or other narcotics in her stomach and intestine, something that we find in the cases of "drug mules." Those are people who are used to transport narcotics inside their bodies, who sometimes die when the capsules rupture in their stomachs, resulting in deadly intoxication. Their bodies might be dismembered to conceal their identities.

After a telephone conversation with the chief of the serology lab, and following his advice, I collect a number of samples for serology tests. In addition to the usual pubic hair and swabs from the vagina and anus, I also take two swabs of the blood that I notice on the chest (especially since I did not have her blood). I also take the spleen (which is good for DNA samples), muscles from the leg and torso, and pieces of bones. To the toxicology lab, I send bile, the gastric contents, and small pieces of the liver, kidney, and spleen.

The case is highly suspicious for homicide, but for today I put the cause of death as "pending" and handle the case as a homicide. I wait for further information from the police investigation and for the toxicology reports on carbon monoxide, drugs, and medication.

The initial information from police is minimal and insufficient: "Subject was decapitated and set on fire. Found by police who observed the fire."

The toxicology report is rushed, and on the same day, I receive results that state the level of carbon monoxide as 3%. That suggests that the woman was dead when her body was set on fire. Later the full results of toxicology come, and the tests do not show any drugs or alcohol. The serology report suggests that her spleen blood is group B. There is no semen on the vaginal or rectal swabs.

As a result of the police investigation, I receive information concerning recent possible crimes, and one case is that of a thirty year old white female who disappeared, according to her husband's report to police. She is the mother of two young children, and she had worked as a secretary of an executive office. The husband is very often the first suspect, so the police carefully continue the investigation. Human blood has been found on number of items received from the apartment of the missing woman: her slippers, a flower vase, a glass music box, a raincoat, the bathtub, washing machine, two sheets, and so on. Further, blood has been found on the samples taken from the family car. Blood and other physiological fluids and tissue contain polymorphic (that is, of various form) genetic markers, such as blood types, which can differ from person to person. These genetic markers are used to compare samples from different sources.

Ten days after the autopsy on the dismembered body, we become convinced that the cause of death is "homicidal violence to head and neck," and we amend the protocol accordingly. We still do not know who she is, and the police still have to find the killer or the killers. The blood sample removed from the chest of the deceased is identified as human blood but without any indication of whose blood it is.

We decide to act from another angle and immediately request medical information on the missing woman. Soon, from a hospital where she has been under examination and treatment, we are sent the x-rays of her left leg. Such luck! Do we not have exactly the same left leg—the one that was left behind in the fire? Right away, we send x-rays, the one from the hospital and another made by us, to an orthopedist from NYU.

Bingo! The orthopedist compares in detail the structure of the separated foot with the hospital's x-ray and confirms the identity. The police take the bad news to the parents. Then, I receive a telephone call from the mother of the deceased. Pain and desperation are in her voice, but she still is very composed. I express my condolences.

She says, "Thank you, doctor. I was informed that it was my daughter, but I still have my doubts. May be it is not her. Maybe she is wandering around somewhere. What else could be done to confirm her identity?"

I call our chief of the serology lab about the mother's concern, asking if anything could be done further for this identification. Remember, this is the early 1990s when our serology laboratory did not do DNA studies routinely (it is later, after September 11, 2001 that we are the most qualified and experienced DNA test center). The chief of serology arranges for the parents' blood and the deceased's blood be studied in a highly qualified private serology center (of course, free of charge for the parents). The results come soon: the parents' and the deceased's blood shows 99.5 % certainty that they are her parents. I call the mother again with this sad but conclusive information. And she is grateful to me for this certainty. Her brain knew that it was her daughter, but her heart refused to believe until it was confirmed.

In a few days, I am called to the grand jury because the husband of the deceased has been arrested for this crime. After so much blood has been found in the apartment, and the body has been identified as that of his wife, the husband confesses to committing the crime. But he does not give any information on how she was killed or whereabouts of her head and the other parts of her body. The case is closed.

"SUICIDE" IN THE HOTEL

In my early days as a medical examiner in the Manhattan office, in addition to performing autopsies we had another duty—to attend the scene of investigation for all cases that were reported to us, including natural deaths, accidental deaths, homicides, and suicides. Once or twice per month, in alternating fashion, all our forensic pathologists participated in this important part of any investigation. It was something new; I had never done it during my one-year fellowship training in the Office of Medical Examiner in Detroit. So, for me it was an interesting experience. I constantly worried about how to do it right, without missing anything important. It looked, though, that I was the only person who worried since none of my colleagues ever expressed any concern. Who knows, maybe growing up as kids with so many crime movies had taught all American doctors something that I had never learned. I kept thinking that crime scenes were supposed to be covered by police detectives who were certainly trained for that work. Anyway, for these and other reasons (such as our work overload, even without this duty), the arrangement did not last long, and the proper organization eventually prevailed.

During our investigative tours, we were going to different parts of the city (Manhattan and the Bronx) with a driver who would remain waiting for us in the car. And there we were, wandering alone, sometimes in a very bizarre situations and places, in civilian clothes with no visible identification. Not all the places in New York were safe and clean, and not all these places looked normal.

Not all the people who lived in these places had normal lives ... but that could be another topic for my stories.

So, on this cold and sunny February day, I was on the investigative tour. When I arrived in a midtown hotel on 47th Street of the West Side, two police detectives were still in the room. On the single hotel bed was a dead body of a thirty-plus year old Hispanic man. The body was in horizontal position and had a slightly bluish face. A pillowcase was tied around the neck with the noose on the left side. The detectives told me that the man had arrived in the hotel the night before and had been found dead in this position by the hotel employee who came to clean the room.

"It looks like a suicide," they told me, pointing to the writing on the bed sheet. The following had been written with a blue pen on the white sheet:

"Dear Police

By the time you read

this I'll be dead on

over dose of drugs

I am sorry but I needed

money so this is what happens

because drugs

I need help and caused trouble in this

World so now I'm dead also

Fight the drug war on

   42 Area"

I did not know why, but some memories inspired by a combination of Sherlock Holms stories and Agatha Christie's books came to mind first. I pushed them off and started to focus on the body lying in the horizontal position, and I started to have my doubts about the suicide. I could not imagine how he managed to hang himself in that position. As a matter of fact, such a conclusion would be wrong because, from forensic pathology textbooks and from my experience, I had learned that people could hang themselves from different positions including horizontal. Nevertheless, with the criminal literature in my mind, I suggested that the detectives check his writing from signing in at the hotel office. I did not know that, in this small midtown hotel, a guest did not have to fill out any papers. At least the photography of the body and the scene were done properly, and the deceased was transported to our morgue for an autopsy the next day.

The case was assigned to me. On the table was the stocky body of a probably Hispanic man with a slightly bluish face and neck and a very obvious one inch wide, pale superficial ligature mark across the neck, from the front to the back. The deceased had several small areas of petechial (pinpoint) bleeding of the sclera and conjunctiva. There were no abrasions or bruises on the neck. Checking his lips, I found lacerations and bruises of the inner surface of the lips and laceration of the inferior lip. The red light! These findings suggested trauma—that somebody applied blunt force to his mouth suppressing his cry for help and his breathing. The suicide assumption became very questionable.

I opened the body, the head, and the neck. In spite of absence of the abrasions and bruises on the neck, the internal examination did show areas of bleeding of the fascia and the neck muscles. Moreover, I found bleeding from the soft tissue of the hyoid bone—the evidence of a possible fracture of the right hyoid bone. And he had the fracture, indeed!

Now, there was no doubt left in my mind: this man had been strangulated by hands (blunt force injury), and a pillowcase was put around his neck immediately after he became unconscious or dead to create a false picture of the suicide. And then the killer wrote the "suicide" note. My diagnosis was "manual strangulation, homicide." I immediately informed the detectives about this outcome.

I did not hear from the detectives for about a month. Then, one day I received the detective's call with the following story. A man in his thirties came to the precinct and talked about drugs in the area and the sad story of his life. He then confessed to the killing, giving the details of the case. He had met the victim in a cheap bar and had been invited to the midtown hotel, where his new acquaintance started sexual advances. He was not homosexual. He needed money, but this unknown man did not want to give him money. So, being stronger and under the influence of drugs, he had strangulated and suffocated the man. Then he put the pillowcase around his neck, wrote the "suicide" note on the sheet, and left the hotel with the little money he had found on the deceased. But now he felt guilt and sorrow ...

I was never called to the trial of the confessed killer.

SERIAL KILLERS

Our society is terrified, puzzled, and even fascinated by an abnormal group of human beings—serial killers. The movie *Dressed to Kill* and "Son of Sam"—remember? Who are serial killers? How and where did they come from? Why they are as they are? What provokes them to be as they are? Could be anything wrong with them genetically? Did they have bad, sadistic childhoods? Was something very wrong with their social life from kindergarten to school or college? Are their brains different? I do not have answers to these questions, and I have never studied the psychology of serial killers. But I never was fascinated or even much interested in these sub-humans, and I did not like the excessive press coverage of their brutal and vicious actions. I personally would deal with them only in the frame of the legal system, according to the law, and I would vote for the death sentence for each and every serial killer.

During my career as medical examiner, I participated twice in the trials of serial killers, both times, of course, as an expert witness.

The Iron Mask Man

Most of my court testimonies were given in New York—in Manhattan, Brooklyn, or the Bronx. But I did occasionally testify in other states. So, one day I received a telephone call from a Manhattan prosecutor about a case that I had done a few years earlier. A young black woman, a dancer in her twenties, had been viciously killed in her dressing room at a nightclub restaurant. Her killer had not been apprehended in New York at that time, but he eventually was arrested in California where he had committed a similar crime. So now I had to go and testify there. The defendant was a serial killer, and quite a few victims of his were from California, as I was told by the prosecutor from Manhattan.

The California trial was supposed to be in Oakland, and I took a direct flight there from New York. I was unlucky and miserable during this flight because my seatmate turned out to be an unbelievably gigantic woman. Her body occupied so much space that, for the six hours of the flight, I could not read, eat, or even move. I was squeezed and crushed by my neighbor. My complaint to the stewardess was to no avail because the flight was full. I felt like a Lilliputian pressed by Gulliver for the whole trip. But the huge woman was comfortable with herself, the food, and my miserable situation. At the Oakland airport, a business car met her, and a police car met me. I might have needed to be met by an ambulance had the flight lasted a bit longer. Very efficiently, with the siren sounding on the way, I was brought half alive to an old-style lakefront hotel in Oakland.

My suite had a bedroom, a conference room, and even a small kitchen. It was very comfortable and luxurious. The windows overlooked an attractive boardwalk along a lake where a few runners could be seen in the warm and pleasant dusk. I wanted to go for a good walk, but I postponed it until the next day, so as to not jeopardize my availability as a witness. Being an experienced New Yorker, I was cautious in that unknown place. After a light supper in the hotel restaurant, I reviewed the autopsy report and went to sleep. Surprisingly, I slept well, and the next morning I awoke fresh and ready for action. The police car promptly came and delivered me (without the siren this time) to the courthouse, but not before I had an excellent cereal and a strong coffee in the cozy old-fashioned hotel restaurant.

The prosecutor, a man in his late thirties, reviewed my

testimony with me. He showed me a stack of newspapers with descriptions of the vicious killings committed by the defendant. The prosecutor surprised me with at least twenty-five portrait-size pictures of the many stab wounds inflicted on the victim from New York. He was ready to present these explicit photos to the jury. Even I was shocked by them, and I expressed my worry about the jury's reaction. In New York, we usually showed slides or prints from slides, but nothing the size of these placards. "It will be okay," the prosecutor reassured me.

My next surprise came when the defendant appeared with his face covered by an iron mask (as in Louis XIV's time!), his hands and feet in shackles. It was not exactly the iron mask of the king's twin brother, but this mask completely covered the defendant's face. It consisted of the set of horizontal metallic strips alternated with transparent plastic; thus, it gave the accused man opportunity to see and hear everything from the courtroom, yet prevented the nasty man from spitting at everyone around him. It was done because the defendant was HIV positive, and he tried to share it with whoever he could.

The defense attorney was sitting unusually quietly a few feet away from his client because, as I was later told, he had stabbed his previous lawyer with a sharp pencil to the chest. The defendant, a young man of around thirty, listened to my testimony carefully without any emotion (as far as I could tell, given the mask) and coldly looked at the portrait-size pictures. With a sense of relief, I finished my testimony and was leaving the courtroom when one member of the jury collapsed during my departure.

The police promptly took me to the airport, and I immediately flew back to New York. My stroll around the picturesque lake did not materialize, and I did not have much opportunity to enjoy my luxury suite. But I was not completely out of luck because on my return flight to New York, I did not have an overweight neighbor. The flight was comfortable, and as always after testifying, I felt relieved. A glass of wine was very appropriate. I read somewhere recently that there may be a change in airline policy for overweight passengers: they may soon be asked to buy two seats on their flights. I do not know if this will be fair to them, and I wonder how the rules will be enforced.

Three years after this trial, I received a telephone call at my Poconos house where I was on a short vacation. The call was from the Oakland detective. He informed me that the next trial would be in Los Angeles where one of the victims of this serial killer was killed.

"What a waste of the taxpayers' money," I thought. But I was never called again about that trial. Might it be that the monster died of AIDS?

A "Friendly" Killer

On a hot night, the eve of Independence Day, a young Hispanic girl was found at a roadside, a hundred feet from the gate to a police range in the Bronx. A vehicle had been observed to stop; a driver had gotten out and walked to the other side of the car. He had opened a passenger door and pulled out something heavy. And then the car had quickly driven away. The body was that of a girl. There were clothes on the upper body, but the body was nude from waist down. There were no identification papers. Several rings and chains were on the girl's neck and hands, and they were vouched by the police.

The next morning, I received the case. The unknown girl, the homicide case ... never easy!

The body was that of a well-developed fifteen to sixteen year old Hispanic girl, five feet, four inches tall, weighing one hundred and five pounds. She was clad in a medium size blue jacket labeled "Jordache Studio," a white and red, a small T-shirt labeled "Fast Turn," a white bra, white socks, and sneakers. As always, a lot of pictures were taken. The Rape Kit was done, and that included head and pubic hair, fingernails, and swabs from the mouth, anus, and vagina.

There were multiple small hemorrhages of the sclera and

conjunctivae—the sign of asphyxia. On the left side of forehead, there was a half inch reddish bruise and also a quarter inch abrasion. On the left cheek and chin there were other half inch abrasions and arc-shaped marks. On the neck, there were two horizontal and parallel ligature marks, going from the front to the back of the neck. A horizontal pattern is usually typical for homicidal strangulation cases, while in cases of hanging, the mark has an upward trend when approaching the back, clearly due to weight of the hanging body. In addition to the ligature marks, there were multiple triangular and arc-shaped (fingernail) marks, irregular linear abrasions, and bruises on the neck. The victim obviously tried to escape the strangulation and fought with the assailant.

There were also abrasions on the chest, abdomen, upper and lower extremities. I did not see any fractures of the neck. I did not see any hemorrhages of the soft tissue, muscles, and fascia of the neck that we see in the victims of manual strangulation and that are usually absent in cases of ligature strangulation. The external genitalia were unremarkable, without any signs of trauma. There was no pregnancy. The internal organs were normal.

As always in our cases, I submitted blood, urine, bile, and small pieces of liver and brain for our toxicology laboratory. For the serology laboratory, I sent blood, head hair, oral, vaginal, and rectal swabs, and fingernails from both hands. The cause of death was obvious: asphyxia due to strangulation by ligature. Manner of death: Homicide.

Within a few days, I received the serology report with positive vaginal and rectal swabs for the presence of semen. There was no semen found in the mouth swabs. The toxicology report was negative for alcohol and drugs. Everything was consistent with rape and homicide.

Several months after the autopsy, I was called as a witness for the trial in the Bronx Court. There, I found that this girl was not the only victim of the killer. As I was told, at least four or five young girls had been found raped and killed in the Bronx, in the same manner, during recent years. The rapist-killer was acquainted with all of them and socialized with their families. For a while, nobody suspected him in the disappearance and killing of their loved ones. The DNA helped to identify the killer.

On the witness stand in the Bronx Court, I presented my findings. In front of me, with the defense lawyer on his right side, sat a handsome Hispanic man in his late twenties or early thirties, with neatly cut and brushed smooth black hair. He wore a dark blue jacket and a white shirt. There was no expression on his face whatsoever, except attentive listening to my testimony of the sexual assault and strangulation. He had mercilessly interrupted the life of the beautiful girl and forever mortally wounded her parents. It was very strange for me to see this good-looking monster, a serial killer, who for a long time was around the families while nobody suspected him of the unbelievable crimes.

He received the life sentence and is still in prison. And we keep paying taxes for his upkeep. He is still alive, and the girls are dead. I do not think that this is fair.

THE "GENERAL'S" NIECE

Once in my early days in the Manhattan office, on a Saturday, I received among three other cases an initially unsuspicious-looking case of a young thirty year old white female. At midnight the night before, the woman had been found on the floor by her boyfriend. EMS had been called, and she had been pronounced dead. The detective passed on information that he obtained from her boyfriend. According to him, the young woman had been depressed over the death of her parents and her brother, and she had spoken about suicide. She was seeing a therapist for her condition. The detective did not see any wounds on the body, and no foul play was suspected.

I performed an autopsy on the white female who appeared to be the stated age of thirty, measured five feet, eleven inches, and weighed one hundred and fifty pounds. Rigidity or stiffness was present. Unfixed libidity also was present on the back. Rigidity and libidity are post mortem events that start immediately after death.

Rigidity is a condition in which muscles of the body become hardened as a result of chemical changes due to lactic acid and other by-products of the tissue metabolism. The process begins at death and usually becomes noticeable within two to four hours, advancing for approximately twelve hours until its completion. It usually starts from the face muscles and proceeds downwards over the body until it stops. The time of the persistence of the rigidity is greatly influenced by the temperature of the body and its environment.

Libidity, also called livor mortis, is a purple discoloration of the skin of depending body parts due to gravity causing the blood to settle into the smallest blood vessels of the skin. The process begins immediately after death. It usually appears after two hours and develops for eight to twelve hours. During this period, if the body is turned over, libidity would shift to the newly dependent areas. That is why we have terms "fixed" and "unfixed" libidity: the purpled discoloration of the skin disappears (blanching) in unfixed libidity and stays unchangeable when it is fixed. Development of libidity also depends on the body and environmental conditions.

It is only in the movies that forensic pathologists or coroners authoritatively pronounce, "She died four hours ago!" In real life cases, we very cautiously give the time range of death because it is always an approximate calculation that depends on many circumstances.

On my further investigation, some petechial hemorrhages, small dots of bleeding, were noticed on the sclera of the eyes. There was a one and a half inch fresh bruise on the left forehead, and there was a one and a half inch bluish bruise on the right anterior thigh.

Upon opening the body and all cavities, I found a three by two centimeter area of bleeding in the soft tissue beneath the above described bruise of the forehead. I also found small petechial hemorrhages of the larynx and bleeding of the soft tissue on the both sides of the chest. (Were they the results of resuscitation?) Her stomach contained a small amount of digested food.

The cause of death was not clear. The case had to be studied much more, and I initially put the cause of death as "pending further study," as we usually do in this kind of case.

When in my office dictating the autopsy, I received a telephone call from the boyfriend of the deceased. On my question of how long he had known the woman, he said about two years. She had worked as the manager of a medical office and was under stress on her job, keeping long hours. Recently, she had complained of tiredness after having the flu two weeks prior. She had been seeing a therapist for two to three years because of the depression that she developed after her mother died. Later all her remaining family members had been killed in a car accident. She had been seeing a psychiatrist but did not need treatment for her depression. She had not been using drugs recently, but seven to eight years prior had "experimented" with cocaine. She had used to take Midol and aspirin. The night before she died, she had had no complaints and felt good. He said he had seen her for the last time at 7:30 am and had talked to her at 5:30 pm on Friday. He had found her on the floor face down and immediately called the EMS; they had come shortly after the call.

"Did they resuscitate her?"

"No, they did not, because she was already dead for five to six hours, as they told me."

This was important information, for me, having in mind the presence of soft tissue bleeding on both sides of the chest. Every occurrence of bleeding that we found on the body had to be explained because it resulted from some blunt force injury to the area of bleeding.

I wanted to talk again with the detective on the case. I wanted to ask his impression of the case and get more details from the scene of the investigation. Yet, I could not find the detective. He had left the precinct for the day after working at night. I decided to see the body again the next morning, a Sunday, because the petechial hemorrhages, a sign of asphyxia, were usually better pronounced with the passing of time. I was sure that the body would remain at OCME, as it had not been cleared yet who would take care of the body.

On the next morning, to my big surprise, I could not find the body. It had disappeared. The funeral home had taken the body. But I did find the detective. I learned again that the case was not under suspicion for homicide, and nothing particular was done during the investigation. I raised my suspicions with the detective. I told him about the presence of soft tissue bleeding of both sides of the chest. I indicated that no resuscitation took place that could have explained these findings. During our conversation, my suspicions were rising higher and higher; I wanted to see the body again that day.

I found that the funeral home was on Long Island. That was not our district and our office area of transportation. I asked the detective, who also started to be nervous and worried, to drive me there to look at the body, and he immediately agreed.

In fifteen minutes, we were driving from our Manhattan office via the Midtown Tunnel and the Long Island Expressway to the Long Island funeral home. Yes, the body was there, and nothing had been done to it yet.

I really was surprised by the amount of the petechial hemorrhages on the deceased's face that had not been that obvious the day before. I wanted to take the body back to our office to see the body again and to show it to other forensic pathologists and to my boss, as well. But the funeral director was not in the area of our office and did not want to transport the body back and forth. On the other hand, I could not to send our transportation to the Long Island funeral home. But I was afraid that I was missing a homicide. When I wrote my personal check for $150 to the Long Island funeral home, the director was persuaded to return the body to the Manhattan office. And it was done!

I looked at the body again making detailed photography of all findings. In addition to the previous findings, I added the presence of middle back bleeding of soft tissue, bilateral areas of soft tissue scapula bleeding, and two bruises of the posterior right thigh. I consulted the case with the chief's deputy who also was working that Sunday, and, the next day, with my boss, the chief medical examiner. As we Russians say, "One head is good, but two are better." After that, the body was returned to the funeral home by the same funeral director. The diagnosis was, of course, still "pending," but I made the toxicology and histology labs rush to exclude any drug overdose or any natural disease as a cause of death. I requested and received the report from the EMS that confirmed the case of no resuscitation.

The toxicology report was negative for any drugs or alcohol. The microscopy of her organs did not reveal anything unusual.

Multiple petechiae on the body and soft tissue bleeding on the both sides of her chest suggested asphyxia as a cause of her death. Her body was pushed and markedly pressed to the floor, causing the bruise on the forehead, and her chest was squeezed from behind by somebody's legs. And after the discussion with my boss, I issued the cause of death, "asphyxia due to compression of neck and chest. Manner: Homicide. How injury occurred: was assaulted by another person."

For a long time, I did not hear anything about this case except for a telephone call from the detective squad sergeant to discuss my diagnosis of the manner of death, because initially no homicide scene investigation was done.

Five years after the autopsy, another detective came to discuss the case with me, and I learned that the young woman was a relative "of a big police boss," and the case was still cold—unresolved. Then after one more year, I received a telephone call from a district attorney who told me about my upcoming testimony on grand jury. The assailant had been apprehended. But I never was called to testify, either because the suspect confessed or the lawyers made a deal. I never learned the outcome. Recently, I decided to find out the outcome of this case. I called the district attorney's office only to discover that the district attorney for this case no longer worked there. My call to the police precinct was also unsuccessful—both detectives had retired and "honestly, the papers could not be found because we had once had a flooding." However, I was satisfied that our findings caused the case to remain open and eventually brought it to some conclusion.

By the way, my $150 was returned to me by the administration of our office.

BODY IN THE TRUNK

A body was found in the trunk of a white Ford Escort in the Bronx. The car was parked on a street near a small park where teenagers liked to play baseball. One of them, when picking up a ball that had hit a nearby car, noticed a bad smell. Another street-smart Bronx kid called it suspicious and brought the car with the smelly trunk to the attention of the police. The car had Connecticut plates.

In the trunk, the Bronx detectives discovered the body of a young white woman. They could not handle this case as anything but as a potential homicide; thus, they immediately bagged both hands of the deceased and took a lot of pictures. The detective at the scene noticed traumatic marks on both the neck and legs. This was not surprising, since the body had been confined in the enclosed space. The body showed strong signs of decomposition.

The first thing the next morning, I performed the autopsy of the woman. An x-ray of the body was done for identification proposes and for exclusion of gunshot wounds. The deceased was wrapped in a blanket stained by decomposed blood. The same stains were present on her T-shirt and her white underwear. A black coat was found separately in the car and was brought to us along with the corpse. All garments were labeled and sent to evidence.

At first I performed the external examination. The deceased was about twenty-three to twenty-five years old, measured five feet, four inches, and weighed one hundred and twenty-eight pounds. Her body showed signs of decomposition with slippage of skin and marbling of the blood vessels. In his book *Medico-legal Investigation of Homicide*, Dr. Werner Spitz said, "The dead body is talking to us." Indeed, just from the first observation I was making my initial impressions. Slippage of the skin and marbling of the vessels were signs of decomposition that suggested it had been around two to three days since her death. But the rate of decomposition, being indicative of the time of death, was also subjected to enormous variations depending on many factors such as the preexisting condition of the body and the temperature in the surrounding space. The body had been found in April, when the nights were cool. The trunk was a confining space, but the woman could have died in a different environment and been put into the trunk sometime later.

Meanwhile, I continued my studies. Fixed libidity on the left side of the body suggested her death had been over twenty-four hours ago. Rigidity, of course, was already absent. An important finding was that multiple intermittent linear abrasions were pointing to marks by ligature on the neck, applied and then released after suffocation. On the right femoral (thigh) area, there was a bluish bruise that could have been there before the assault. The same I could say about the brownish abrasions of the left lower extremity. On the third finger of the left hand, there was a linear abrasion. I concluded my external examination by taking the rape kit that included head and pubic hair, fingernails, and swabs from the mouth, anus, and vagina. Multiple photos of the body were made.

Then I performed the internal examination. Upon opening the neck, there was bleeding of the left muscle, bleeding of the soft tissue above the thyroid cartilage, and bleeding around both ends of hyoid bone. There were no fractures, but fractures of the hyoid bone were a rare event for young people dying of strangulation. Further, the tongue revealed areas of bleeding. Other internal organs were unremarkable. The woman was not pregnant. Small pieces of internal organs and traumatic areas were taken for microscopic study. Toxicology material was taken to the lab. A postmortem dental examination was done by our forensic dentist—important in this case for identification of the unknown female.

All these findings, including petechial hemorrhages of the sclera, conjunctivae, and larynx, hemorrhages of the soft tissue of the thyroid and hyoid bone, congestion and multiple abrasions of the neck, and bleeding of neck muscle on the left side, suggested that strangulation was done by combined force of hands as well as ligature. Thus, upon completion of the autopsy, I issued the cause of death: "Strangulation. Manner: Homicide."

The post-autopsy tests did not contradict the final conclusion. Toxicology showed that the deceased did not have any drugs. Only 0.1 % alcohol was revealed, and that could be either the result of digested alcohol before death or of decomposition. The microscopic study of the internal organs did not reveal any abnormality. The rape kit was negative, but semen was found in condom number one (of the two condoms brought to the lab directly by the police detective from the scene). The police investigation identified the young woman as a missing resident of Connecticut. Her identity was established by her mother and confirmed by a dental report.

I did not hear anything about the case for two and half years until I received a subpoena to testify in the Superior Court of Connecticut, meaning that the investigation was completed and the charges were brought.

The prosecutor of the case gave me a call and discussed my findings and conclusions, but very briefly, not longer than for fifteen minutes. He informed me that, according to investigators, the woman had been seen having a dinner with her boyfriend between 5:30 pm and 7:00 pm two days before her body was found in the Bronx.

"Is that consistent with the findings?" asked the prosecutor.

"Yes, it is. Everything depends on the environmental conditions that the body was subjected to after death. The degree of decomposition is indicative of timing between two to three days. But if her dead body was kept at a warm temperature, decomposition could develop much earlier; and if she was seen alive approximately forty-eight hours before finding her, it is not impossible."

The prosecutor arranged the day and the time of my testimony and informed me that an inspector would come and drive me to the prosecutor's office and then to the court. It was very nice because I wouldn't have to drive myself from Manhattan to the courthouse in another state.

The next day, after my conversation with the prosecutor, the defense attorney called me. He did not question the cause of death—it was obvious—but his theory was that the death was accidental. I definitely could not resolve this issue because I only see and testify about all the signs of strangulation that caused the deceased's asphyxia. I could not clarify if it was applied intentionally or accidentally. This was the business of defense and prosecution. By the way, I liked the defense lawyer because he spent much more time on discussion of the case than the prosecutor. Every sign on the dead body—rigidity, libidity, decomposition, slippage of skin, and the greenish discoloration—were discussed in detail. We spent more than a whole hour on this discussion. He did his homework and definitely was going to be prepared for his defense.

Soon came the day of my testimony. The inspector, a tall, fit police officer in his late thirties, took me from my apartment in New York, and after about a fifty-minute drive, we were in the court building of Stamford, Connecticut. My meeting with the prosecutor was very short again, but I still managed to inform him about my long discussion with the defense attorney who had legitimate interest in the postmortem changes that could be for and against his defense. The prosecutor, though, remained confident with no reaction whatsoever to my warnings.

On the stand, as many times before, I was in front of the jury, the prosecutor, the defense lawyer, and the defendant, who happened to be the dead woman's boyfriend with whom she wanted to break her relationship. He was a dark-haired man in his late twenties wearing a dark blue suit and white shirt. There were two police officers behind him. In spite of my many and frequent testimonies, I could not stop wondering when I saw the non-emotional face of the defendant. What was in his mind? What did he feel? Why did he do that, and how did he manage to show nothing?

The prosecutor asked me to describe my findings concerning the cause of death. He was short and precise in his questions. It did not take much time to finish my testimony with him. Then, I was questioned by the defense attorney who methodically discussed every detail of the body and each sign of decomposition. The jury listened attentively to his questions and to my answers. We did not finish before lunch time, and we had a break. Because I was still on the stand and under the oath and did not know anybody in this unfamiliar place, I silently had my coffee and chewed a small toast in the nearby coffee-shop. Then, the defense resumed the questioning. I thought that he would never finish it; he repeated the same questions again and again. I understood that it was his strategy. He knew that the jury already might have forgotten that she was killed by strangulation. The terms that were unfamiliar to them and the uncertain timeframe in relation to the events might have created doubts about the guilt of the defendant.

The result of the trial was a mistrial. So much about trial games!

After a few months, I received a new subpoena and was ready to testify again. But fortunately, it was not necessary: the defendant pleaded guilty.

"So he did do it!" was my thought.

***

This case was suspicious from the very beginning because the body was found in a trunk; therefore, it had to be put there by somebody. Decomposition did not significantly obscure the findings and interpretation of the cause of death, so the diagnosis was straightforward immediately after the autopsy. But it was not so obviously simple in another of my cases when a body, with signs of decomposition, was found at home. Decomposition itself might create changes that could be similar to those caused by strangulation and resulting in asphyxia: bulging eyes, a protruding tongue, and discoloration of the neck muscles.

I recall the case that I had in 1987, only my second year with OCME. At the time, I was working in the Brooklyn office. It was my busy day, with three cases on hand. One of them was a teenager of seventeen with a stab wound to abdomen, another, a ten year old boy who hung himself, and the third was the case of a twenty-four year old woman found dead and already decomposed on the floor of her apartment. On autopsy of this third case, I did not see any signs of trauma. She did have severe decomposition—her eyes were bulging, her tongue had protruded through her mouth. She had two arc-shaped very superficial reddish abrasions on the neck. Upon opening her neck, I did not find any fractures of the hyoid bone or thyroid cartilage. The right side of her neck muscle was reddish, but, of course, that could have been a result of decomposition. I made pictures of all these findings, and put temporary conclusions as: pending further study, CUPPI, which is, circumstances unclear, pending police investigation. I was suspicious of asphyxia as the cause of her death. But of course, it was important first to have the police investigation and the toxicology report for drugs and medication in her system. The toxicology report came back negative. I still did not release the case, but waited for the new report from the detective. And the detective did call me soon with the information that she was strangulated, according to the confession of her boyfriend to his father! Then, I received a call from the district attorney with the same information and a question of whether my findings were consistent with this new revelation. I said, "Yes, they are." The case was finalized, the cause of death: strangulation. Homicide.

From such not obvious cases with mild signs of asphyxia yet with marked signs of decomposition, we learn and gain our experience and substantiate our intuition based on such experience and facts. Forensic pathologists' intuition is not congenital. It is acquired.

THE TEENAGER FROM NEW ENGLAND

"At the above location the subject was found unresponsive in the apartment where she was staying with another druggy that she befriended. The subject is a runaway, partially dressed. The subject was found in bed face up. The room was filled with condoms and glassine envelopes. The case is being held as a noncriminal death at this time. There were no signs of a struggle, and the property of the apartment was intact."

I received this report from our OCME detective who, in turn, had received the information from the assigned detective of the precinct of this location. I talked with the precinct detective on the telephone, and he added that the girl was found on a bed with a lot of exudate fluid around her nose and mouth.

"It looks as overdose," was his opinion.

There were no witnesses. The owner of the apartment "had a bad feeling about this girl and called 911 to check on her. Police and EMS came and discovered the girl dead in her bed."

Our medical investigator, who went to the scene the same day, added to this information that the girl was found in the rear bedroom of the first floor apartment. The door of the apartment was closed but not locked. The apartment was insecure, and drug paraphernalia was present. The scene was pronounced as a crime scene, and all normal procedures were followed. The deccased did not rent the apartment; rather it was rented to her associate. Her associate had been arrested a few months before for bringing females from New England to New York for prostitution.

The deceased was found partially clothed. Rigor mortis (post mortem stiffing of the body) was present on the head, neck, and extremities. Livor mortis (postmortem discoloration of the body) was purple, mostly fixed in the areas corresponding to the body position. No signs of trauma were noted on external examination at the scene.

I performed the autopsy the next morning. The deceased wore only an orange dress shifted basically to the chest area; she also had an orange band on the right femoral area and a black band on the right wrist. Her hands were covered by paper bags due to suspicion of homicide. The left side of the face and part of the right cheek, near the nose, were bluish. There was a consolidated one-eighth inch diameter hemorrhage of the left sclera. In the middle of the nose, there was a one-eighth inch reddish abrasion. On the left side of the nose, there was a one-fourth by one-half inch linear abrasion with a surrounding bluish area. The tip of the nose was pale with a horizontal reddish abrasion above the pale area. The nostrils had marginal reddish abrasions. Beneath the nose, bilaterally, there were reddish abrasions of about one-half inch by one-half inch. Beneath these abrasions, near the mouth, there was a horizontal whitish area of one-fourth inch width. No injury to the mouth was observed.

The following internal examination did not reveal anything significant to be considered as the cause of her death. The girl was not pregnant. She did not have any trauma except the abrasions on her face, described above. A number of pictures were taken by our photographer. I took the rape kit for the serological study. An x-ray of the head was done, and later I discussed it with the radiologist who excluded any fractures, particularly a nose fracture. I took blood, bile, urine, and small pieces of internal organs for toxicology to study drugs, alcohol, and medication in her system. And of course, I sent material to the histology lab for studies of the internal organs. I also requested more information from the police detective, the so called DD5 form. For the time being, I put the cause of death as "pending further study," handling this case as a homicide.

The girl was recognized by a relative with the help of pictures and from the tattoo on her shoulder. She was identified as a missing sixteen-year-old from one of the New England states. The toxicology was rushed after the autopsy, and the report I received indicated that she had small amounts of methadone in her blood and nothing else. The histology of her internal organs was normal.

I discussed the case with my two bosses, the chief medical examiner and the deputy of my branch. We all arrived in agreement that the cause of her death was "asphyxia by covering of the nose and mouth. Manner: Homicide."

I had never been called to a grand jury or trial and had not heard anything about further developments on this case. Nothing unusual for us—it meant either the case was still open, or it was settled. When writing this sad story, I decided to try a computer search for any public information about this case, and I found some.

There was a news article stating that this New England state had an 11% higher than average narcotics usage, and marihuana was a drug of choice for its youngsters. They were not aware of the danger of this drug that actually can be a step toward other hard drugs—cocaine and heroine. The suffocation homicide death in New York of the sixteen year old girl was mentioned as an example of a case involving cocaine and heroin drug traffic along with prostitution. There was no information on whether anybody was arrested and prosecuted in the death of the girl.

Well, this is not a fiction story, and I cannot create a happy ending. It would not be happy, even in the event of an apprehension in the case. This is life with no simple solution. Of course, in my practice of forensic pathology, I witnessed a lot of resolved cases, where criminals were found, tried, and punished. Being a forensic pathologist and an expert witness on grand juries and/or at trials, I must objectively present my findings. My conclusions have to be based on 100% proof and not on hypotheses or fantasies. We, forensic pathologists, are not concerned with who was the killer or killers. It is the role of the prosecution to prove the evidence of the guilt of the defendant. I vividly remember one case where the prosecutor was certain that the deceased was killed by the person who was on trial as a defendant. The case ended as a mistrial. Later, talking with the prosecutor, I was surprised to learn that she was actually glad of this outcome because, as it turned out, another person had committed the crime. There is nothing worse than convicting an innocent person!

KARATE CASE

In the late 1980s, shortly after I started working in the Manhattan office, we were severely overloaded with cases, and many of them were serious and time consuming. It was a great relief to no longer be alone in New York, as my husband Sam had joined me in our one-bedroom apartment. He had found a newly open position at Long Island's high technology robotic firm. So, I had now somebody to complain to about my tough and overwhelming job. It's a good thing that Sam got used to the specifics of my specialty as a forensic pathologist and could stand the details, sometimes quite gruesome, as told during our dinners together.

It was on one of those days, when I had three autopsies: the case of a fifty year old woman who sustained multiple injuries as a hit-by-car pedestrian, the case of a thirty-two year old woman who had drowned in the bathtub with an alcohol level of 0.48 (very drunk!), and the case of a twenty-four year old young man who was assaulted and later on died in the hospital. This definitely sounded like homicide, and my attention was drawn to it.

Initial information from the hospital suggested that the young man had been kicked in the chest and had fallen back and struck his head on pavement. He was admitted to the hospital unconscious. A CT-scan had been performed and showed a large area of subarachnoid (the space between two soft layers of the protective brain tissue) bleeding. The electrocardiogram showed no activity. Three days after the admission to the hospital, he was pronounced dead. The police gave me additional information that the young man was struck to the chest or neck by the assailant who used his boot in the swift and single hit that caused the young man's immediate fall and unconsciousness.

I was dealing with this case as we usually did with the cases of homicide: x-rays, photography, sending blood, scalp, pubic hair, and clipped nail samples to the serology lab. On external examination, the body revealed no obvious injury except for two quarter inch, purple-bluish bruises, one linear and one round, on the right side of the chest. On the anterior left arm, there were four linear vertical abrasions, one to two inches in length.

The subsequent autopsy revealed extensive subarachnoid hemorrhage. There were no fractures. There were no contusions of the brain. And there was no aneurysm rupture, a very common cause of such bleeding. However, on the neck, in the vicinity of the right carotid artery and the jugular vein, there was a two and a half centimeter area of hemorrhage of the fascia and soft tissue that covered the right carotid artery and right jugular vein. It might have been the area of impact. Upon opening the posterior surface of the neck, I found a one centimeter by one and a half centimeter hemorrhage of the soft tissue of the right side that definitely looked like the continuation of the same area of the suspected impact. I checked with the hospital to see if any injections were performed in this area. The answer was negative. Both lungs showed marked consolidation of all lobes, the evidence of bronchopneumonia (lung inflammation). The young man had survived three days in the hospital, and this was the usual complication of anoxic encephalopathy (lack of oxygen in the brain) and coma in an unconscious man.

I certified the death as "head trauma with subarachnoid hemorrhage sustained during assault. Manner: Homicide."

Nobody had been arrested yet, but newspapers were full of information. We, of course, did not base our diagnosis on the newspapers. The police detectives had to investigate this case of homicide thoroughly in order to present it to the district attorney. The police were looking for a young man who had worn a green beret when he delivered the powerful spin kick to the deceased.

The newspapers related the very sad and tragic story of the victim, full of life and energy, who celebrated his birthday with friends and who happened to be in the wrong place at the wrong time with the other group of the young men. Moreover, the deceased was portrayed as a peacemaker trying to reduce a confrontation that cost him his life. The assailant had fancy boots that probably were a subject of the joke that caused the confrontation, and he had used a boot for the karate-kick that fatally injured the victim. The suspect was believed to be a karate expert, and the detectives were trying to track him by checking karate schools. They were also tracking ballet dancers who could produce similar damage with their legs.

I did not have any knowledge of the injuries that could be produced with karate, and there was not much literature about it. But I learned that the word karate was derived from the Japanese symbol meaning empty hand. Within the past decades, karate had been encouraged as a competitive sport. At that time, I think, almost every family thought that it had to be a part of their children's physical education. I do not like karate and always remember this very tragic case. I am always against it as a sport for children. In spite of my opinion, all my grandchildren have had these lessons, and some advanced from belt to belt. The reason, as my sons explained to me, was that the children were busying themselves with this very useful (?!) exercise for self-defense and for the development of coordination and discipline.

So, what I learned about karate was really frightening. The hand of the karateka, or expert in karate, can develop a peak velocity of ten to fourteen meters per second and exert a force of more than three thousand newtons (that translates to six hundred and seventy-five pounds). In various kicks, the foot reaches speeds of between seven to fourteen meters per second (*The Physics of Karate* by M.S. Feld, et al.). The karateka applies a large amount of momentum to a small area of his opponent's body. It is enough to break wooden blocks and concrete, not to mention tissue and bone.

I am not fond of films with karate action and fighting and really do not clearly remember watching any of the famous Bruce Lee movies. But maybe I did see some of them, because in my mind they kept very professional with iron discipline and decency in using this dangerous and powerful form of the martial arts only in righteous situations against evil forces. Unfortunately, new practitioners of karate sometimes forget one of the traditional karate rules: the karateka must be not only a person of excellent physical discipline, but also of mental discipline. In a forensic pathology textbook by Adelson, it is stated that blunt traumata are caused by the force produced by mass and acceleration (F=MA) and that the degree of injury depends on the rate at which energy is liberated and the size of the impact area. This makes the injuries produced by a karateka especially severe and dangerous.

Was the finding of the autopsy consistent with karate used as a weapon? Yes, it was. There was no indication of other causes which might have actually killed the victim. The only finding suggesting the blunt force injury impact was the hemorrhage of the soft tissue of the neck. As the result of this impact, the young man had a grave internal injury—subarachnoid bleeding—that killed him. The detailed report of our neuro-pathologist confirmed the autopsy finding. The brain had massive subarachnoid hemorrhage of traumatic origin. There was no aneurysm anywhere. A blood clot was densely adherent to the right vertebral artery. An examination of the cervical spine revealed no hemorrhage in or around the vertebral arteries up to the dissected level.

***

The twenty-one year old suspect who tried to escape from New York was arrested twelve days after the assault. He was charged with second degree murder and manslaughter and was indicted by grand jury. The trial was months after the assault. The team of the private forensic pathologists and neuropathologists requested and examined all our findings, reports, and all material that we had in possession in the Office of Chief Medical Examiner. Their main goal was to check for anything that could make the death unavoidable, such as the presence of a congenital abnormality—for example, a brain vessel aneurysm that caused the fatal bleeding—or anything that was not properly done during the autopsy or in our investigation of the case. They found nothing different from what our office did.

There was a trial of the young, blonde-haired man who had killed the innocent young man and forever destroyed the life of his devastated parents. The victim's parents were present at this trial. As an expert witness, I testified about injury and the cause of his death. I was not present on the other testimonies. I really never knew the details of the proceedings. I just know that it is not so easy to kick somebody with a boot to the neck. You have to be trained in this swift, strong leg movement, reaching the other body so high. The defendant was convicted to four years in prison.

Around twenty years passed, and when I was writing my stories, I made some computer searches and was amazed to find more to the sad story. The parents of the victim established memorial funds, and symposiums took place at the college where the young man graduated. It was a very good memorial.

CHILD ABUSE

When I told one of my colleagues that I was writing some tales of a forensic pathologist, she exclaimed, "Don't you have enough of it?!"

What she meant was that for years and years we dealt with the terrible stories of human life—viciousness without borders, the senseless deaths of beautiful people, the pain of parents losing their children, human misery, and other irreversible tragedies. But by far the worst in my experience were the cases of child abuse where parents killed their helpless children. I have always thought that these people deserve the death penalty. There is absolutely no excuse and forgiveness for them in my mind. The same colleague, after seeing my persistent intention to write my stories, said, "Well, it is apparently a treatment," and she was most likely right.

During my long carrier as a forensic pathologist, I performed autopsies on multiple cases involving child abuse. I encountered them more frequently than people might think. Here I have selected a few to paint the picture.

The Panhandler

It was a cold January day in New York City. On the corner of Second Avenue and 28th Street, near a garbage can full of empty boxes, old newspapers, empty bottles, and pieces of food, a skinny Hispanic man in his thirties was standing and holding to a gray worn down stroller. He stood there in an old shabby coat, a small ski-hat barely covering his black curly hair. He had dirty, white socks overhanging his run-down shoes. He did not have any gloves, and his hands were bluish red. He was unkempt with few days' of beard stubble on his face. His lifeless, dark eyes looked pitifully at every pedestrian who crossed the street. His left hand was outstretched toward the people passing by, and his right hand was on the baby stroller. He begged for himself and his child. Apparently the child was covered by an old, red blanket, but because of the stroller hood, the head and face of the child could not be seen. The hurried people did not pay much attention to the unusual beggar with the child. In those years in New York, there were plenty of beggars at this part of the city. Accustomed to everything, New Yorkers kept rushing to work with no visible surprise or other emotions. But one Good Samaritan, a man in his middle thirties, stopped near the panhandler, gave him money, and tried to see the hidden child. The child was motionless and pale and did not look to be sleeping. A red bruise was obvious on her cheek. He said, "You must go immediately to the hospital! I will pay for the cab."

He stopped a cab, gave the driver money, and asked the cabbie to take the child and the man to the closest hospital. The man did not resist. The Good Samaritan was on his way as soon as the cab moved. The man was brought to the New York Medical Center where his girl was pronounced dead on arrival. The doctors immediately called the cops who arrested the man. The Office of Medical Examiner received the child's body, and I was assigned to the case.

She was a tiny, three year old black child, measuring three feet, four inches and weighing only thirty pounds. On her right cheek, there was a doughnut-shaped purple bruise, three quarters of inch in diameter. The left cheek also had several purple bruises up to a half inch in diameter. On the left side of the forehead there was a one inch by one inch bluish discoloration, and on the lower part of the chest and abdomen there were multiple pinkish and bluish bruises from a quarter inch to a half inch in diameter.

On the back and buttocks of the body, there were the same size bruises and one scar, a half inch long. On the left lower extremity, there was another half inch scar.

In addition to these multiple bruises and scars, the child's body was covered by multiple punctuated lesions on the face, head, chest, abdomen, and upper and lower extremities. They were in different stages of healing. Some had a crust, and some others had already lost it. It reminded me the highly contagious children's infection—the varicella (chickenpox) that I had dealt with in my pediatric practice shortly after graduation from medical school. But combined with the multiple bruises they looked more ominously as traumatic lesions that might be present in the case of an obviously abused child.

Upon the opening the skull, I found there were no fractures. Multiple hemorrhages of the soft tissue were beneath the described bruises of the head. The brain had severe edema and many small foci of subarachnoid (soft capsule) bleeding. Inside the chest, beneath the bruise, there was bleeding of the soft tissue of the anterior seventh and eighth ribs, but there were no fractures. Upon opening the abdominal cavity, I found four hundred and fifty milliliters of blood. The internal surface of the abdominal wall, corresponding to the abdominal bruises, had areas of bleeding. On the lower surface of the liver, there was a two centimeter by one centimeter laceration, and that had been the origin of the abdominal bleeding. Also, the small intestine had areas of bleeding and small lacerations of the mesentery (that is, the membranous folds attaching the small intestine to the body wall).

I was handling this as a homicide case. Prior to the autopsy, x-rays were done to exclude old and recent fractures, and none were found in this child. Our professional photographer was doing pictures of the whole body with particular attention to the injuries. I was taking material for the toxicology lab to study drugs, medication, and alcohol in the blood and other tissue. I sent blood samples to the Health Department lab to exclude my suspicion for varicella, and I sent the serology lab samples of blood, scalp hair, and anal, vaginal, and oral swabs for the exclusion of sexual assault. Saliva from a suspicious bite mark bruise on the right cheek was also sent to serology. And as always, small pieces of internal organs were taken for histology to check for typical childhood diseases. In cases of child abuse, the injuries must be studied for age. Because of this, the injured organ areas and spots of bleeding of the soft tissue were taken for microscopy.

Based on multiple bruises of different parts of the body, bleeding of the brain capsule and the soft tissue of the left rib, lacerations of the liver and mesentery of the small bowel, and the four hundred and fifty milliliters of blood in the abdominal cavity, I put the cause of death as blunt force injuries to the head and abdomen with liver and mesentery lacerations and internal bleeding. Manner: Homicide.

Multiple bruises of the body suggested that the child was beaten many times. This girl with her weight of thirty pounds had about nine hundred milliliters of blood in her body. She had lost 50 % of her total blood. The child did not die immediately after the beating. It could have taken hours because the bleeding from the liver and the mesentery was slow. It was not arterial bleeding, which usually flows fast. The child could have been suffering for hours, gradually losing consciousness, and nobody brought her for help. The punctuated skin lesions, as I suspected already on autopsy, were indeed lesions of varicella. That was confirmed by the immunological study by the Health Department. She had had this varicella for one to three weeks. But of course, this was not the cause of her death

The newspapers published a lot of information about the family. The panhandler was arrested and charged with murder. He was a Cuban refugee who lived with the girl's mother and her other three children in a hotel for the poor that the city provided for homeless families. The girl was not his daughter. Hotel tenants claimed that the couple smoked crack regularly, and one of the tenants told police that she often sold crack to this man and his girlfriend. Actually, the last time she had sold them crack had been on the day the child was taken to the hospital. The day before, the mother had given birth to another baby, a son of the Cuban refugee panhandler. Still unnamed, that baby was in another hospital being monitored for signs of the drug withdrawal.

According to a city official close to this case, "his family itself has been known to us for a long time." Social services officials admitted that they had been "actively investigating the family of the three-year-old when she was being battered to death." It was a tragedy, but disaster was waiting. And this woman had just given birth to another child! A spokeswoman for the Human Resources Administration said that there "was no prior indication of abuse in this dead girl's case."

This case happened in the late 1980s, and many good things have been done since that time, but unfortunately the child abuse cases have not disappeared, and, no doubt, much more must be done in the system.

Little Tracy

Tracy was born prematurely with low weight and with heart problems. Shortly after birth, she was abandoned by her mother. The little girl was transferred to one of the good New York hospitals where she was kept for three months, gaining her weight and height. The hospital personnel loved this tiny, smiling baby girl. They were very pleased that she would be with the foster family who took her from the hospital.

The foster mother was a registered nurse who was married to a physical therapist, and Tracy was with them for nine months. She did what every normal baby would—learned sitting on her small buttocks or standing in her bed strongly holding to the wooden frame. She smiled proudly to her adoptive parents showing them her three teeth. She ate cereals, tried and liked fruits and vegetable dishes, and drank milk and juices. Tracy was a happy, lovely child with huge black eyes and soft curly hair nicely surrounding her round face.

But the social workers were looking for another foster parent couple, a black one, because Tracy was black, and the registered nurse and her husband were white. So, a very nice black couple was found who took Tracy home and, after couple of months, decided to adopt her.

During these months of care, the foster mothers reported that the natural mother did not show any interest in her baby and that she ignored court summonses, letters, and personal contacts regarding the baby. But all of a sudden, the natural mother demanded the girl, and in spite of the protests of both foster families, a family court judge sent the eighteen month old girl back to her mother.

Several months later, Tracy was brought by ambulance to the hospital for difficulties in breathing. On arrival the child had multiple bruises and an old burn on her left palm. An x-ray showed possible pneumonia. Unfortunately, within minutes of arrival the child was pronounced dead. The hospital doctors felt that the child was abused due to the multiple bruises and scars on her body. The mother admitted to striking the child with a rubber tube. Thus, the child's body was sent to our Office of Medical Examiner.

As usual, I performed the external and internal examinations after the x-ray of the whole body was done. She was of normal height and weight and had multiple bruises, abrasions, and scars everywhere, including the face. Some of them were recent bruises. On the forehead, there were two bluish bruises one-and-quarter-inch in diameter, multiple small abrasions in the area of the right eye, a bluish bruise near the right eyebrow, a bluish discoloration of the left temple measuring one and a quarter inch in diameter, superficial abrasions of the tip of the nose and nostrils and the upper lip, and an abrasion of the left cheek—all of these painted a very grim picture. And that was not all: there were duplicate arch-shaped, half inch abrasions on the chest and similar ones on the palm. On the right and left upper extremities, the buttocks, and the back, there were multiple healing and fresh abrasions, bruises, and long and short scars.

Upon the opening the skull, I found there was a hemorrhage in the soft tissue of the area corresponding to the bruise on the left temple. My examination revealed a left subdural hematoma, bleeding under the outermost brain capsule, with fifty gram blood clots, plus a subarachnoid hemorrhage, that is, bleeding of the soft vascular capsule of the brain. The lungs showed small areas of consolidation suspicious for pneumonia. The latter was confirmed by microscopic study. The x-ray study by our radiologist revealed a deformity of the forearm bone, thus indicating a healed greenstick fracture.

The child had subdural hematoma as the result of a blunt force injury to the head. A blow inflicted with an open hand to the face or head may cause subdural hematoma. Multiple bruises and abrasions of different sizes and age were suggestive of repetitive beating. I concluded that this was a child abuse case—a homicide.

Tracy's mother was arrested and charged with murder. One and half years after the child's death, she stood in front of the judge at family court. She did not deny beating the child with electrical wire. Her other four children were placed in the care of the city welfare officials—a procedure that is always done in the case of child abuse.

So many mistakes were made in the management of this child! The foster mothers were denied the right to testify when the decision was made to return Tracy to her mother. The mother's indifference to the baby was also ignored. The child was returned to her mother with suggestions of frequent social worker visits that never took place. A social worker visited the family only once—long before Tracy's death. Then she left the job, and no one continued the visit. Tracy's mother was a battered woman who had been in a shelter for battered women, and battered women are known as the highest risk for battering children. And in the months before Tracy's death the social worker visited the family only once?! The dead child's father was listed in court documents with "address unknown." It always infuriated me when only women were accused in abusing children. In fact, according to the family, after "a big fight," this man put Tracy's mother out on the winter street with a week-old baby—another one that she just had by C-section. Not long after that, the family court judge ordered Tracy's return to her mother. The mother's family had found an apartment for her and her children. They did not have food. They begged for food from neighbors. Mistakes, mistakes, mistakes—and the child is dead.

"Are you pleading guilty to manslaughter of the second degree?" the clerk asked in the family court.

"Yes."

The judge, in accepting the plea bargain, said that the mother's "volatile conduct stemmed from a mental disease." He said he would consider probation if her lawyers found a proper mental health residence. Tracy's mother was free to leave. By the way, the father was supposed to pay for Tracy's funeral. This was the last time that Tracy's mother heard of him. She said, "He ran away with the money for burying the baby."

Lethal Bathing

An eight month old Hispanic child, Pedro, was in the bathtub with his brother, two year old Santo. It was a routine procedure for finishing a day for the two very active brothers. They looked so nice and clean with their smoothed, black hair and dark, shiny eyes. After bathing, they slept much better in their separate little beds. There was no father in their very modest one-bedroom apartment at the eighth floor of the project building because the boys' twenty-two year old single mother was raising her two children on welfare.

The telephone rang, and the mother left the children in the bathtub, as she frequently did. She got involved in talking with her sister, arguing about issues which bothered both of them. Then a little distracted by the conversation, she started cleaning the living room of the many toys spread around the floor by her children. She noticed the older boy appearing in the room, taking his toy truck and returning to the bathroom. All of a sudden, he gave a desperate cry, "Mama!" She immediately ran to the bathroom and discovered her little eight month old baby floating in the water face down.

The mother called 911 and while waiting for EMS started chest compression by following instructions for resuscitation. When the EMS brought the child to the hospital, he was in full cardiopulmonary arrest. They continued resuscitation efforts, but with no success, and a half-hour after admission, the child was pronounced dead. The hospital sent the child's body to the Office of Medical Examiner. The mother objected to the autopsy, but we explained to her that the autopsy had to be done, and her objection could not be accepted.

I performed the autopsy the same day we received the body, following the night that the child had died in the hospital. He was a good child with normal weight and height. Nothing unusual was found on external examination. But internal examination revealed a two centimeter by two centimeter bleeding of the soft tissue of the left lateral skull. There was also a healing fracture six centimeters in length in the same area, the left parietal bone. The brain showed edema. All other organs were unremarkable.

Bleeding of the soft tissue and the healing fracture of the skull suggested a blunt force injury to the head that took place prior to the drowning in the bathtub. From our detective and from the district attorney, who was immediately involved with the child's death, I received information that three weeks prior, the child had fallen from the bed. The mother had not gone immediately to the doctor. Only after five days, when the baby had seizures, did she take him to a doctor, who made an x-ray and diagnosed the fracture of the skull. The BCW (the children's protection agency) responded right away with a home visit, but found nothing wrong. It is very unusual for children under five to have a fracture of the skull after falling from the bed. But because there was no other indication of child abuse at the time of injury, the event was accepted as consistent with the fall. No treatment was prescribed, and, according to the mother, the child was normal all this period.

It was different this time. The cause of death was:

1. Drowning; left unattended.
2. Healing blunt force head injury with skull soft tissue bleeding and left parietal fracture. Brain edema.

The manner of death: Homicide.

Small children must not be left alone in a bathtub with water in it. It is negligence. When it results in death, it is homicide because the death is caused by the action of the other person, the mother in this case. I could not exclude that the child might have had a seizure being in the bathtub after the head trauma. He already had a history of seizures. That was another important reason to not leave the child unattended.

Thus, negligence after negligence in this case led to child's death. I was not called to testify in the family court, as frequently happened in other cases. Perhaps the case was settled with a plea bargain for a lesser charge.

Acute Heroin Intoxication

Acute drug intoxication is a very common diagnosis in our practice as a cause of death of young and otherwise healthy people who have been drug-users. The case of a little child was unusual, unexpected, and very sad. A three year old child was brought to a hospital from his home dead on arrival. According to parents, he refused to eat breakfast and lunch that day. The only history of child's diseases was chickenpox, two weeks prior.

I performed an autopsy on the black child, age three, with

multiple healing lesions of chicken pox. I did not see any signs of trauma, and all internal organs looked grossly normal. There were no congenital abnormalities. After the autopsy, it still was not clear why the child had died. I saved the brain for neuropathology study, and I took blood, bile, urine, the contents of the stomach, and small pieces of the liver, brain, and kidneys for toxicology studies for drugs and medication. I took blood and a stool culture for a microbiology study, and I requested more a detailed police report.

Microscopic study of all the internal organs did not reveal anything unusual. The blood culture just showed some postmortem contamination by bacteria. But the toxicology report revealed opiates in the blood, brain, and urine. And quite a lot! The child had heroin in his system, and that was the cause of his death. Immediately, I informed the police, and their investigation found heroin presence and usage by one of the parents. The child had found the heroin container and consumed the contents.

In the death certificate, I put the cause of death: acute opiates intoxication. Manner: Homicide. Why homicide?—because it was criminal negligence of the parents and because the child's death was inflicted by the illegal actions of the others. I do not know how the parents were punished by the system, but I do know that they had already punished themselves severely.

DROWNING IN THE BATHTUB

Adult drowning in a bathtub is often a complicated medical/legal problem. It usually is a result "of unconsciousness brought by disease (epilepsy, heart disease) or after consumption of alcohol and/or drugs," as our forensic textbook states. Of course, I had quite a few such cases, and I would like to describe three of them, showing the controversy that can arise in their interpretation.

A twenty-one year old black female was found in a bathtub filled with water. She was fully dressed in a black shirt, white jeans, black bra, white underwear, and white socks. Rigidity was absent and libidity was unclear. On the face and knees, she had slippage of skin. On the forehead, there were multiple small linear horizontal abrasions, and a half-inch laceration with a bruise. Both feet and hands had the typical appearance of washerwoman skin (wrinkling of the skin) due to prolonged immersion in water.

Upon opening the skull, I saw bleeding of the soft tissue of the skull beneath the abrasions, bruise, and laceration. She also had bleeding of the soft tissue of the skull on the back of her head. These findings suggested to me that blunt force injury took place at the front and back (blows), and not once but twice. She did not have fractures of the skull, and this suggested that the blows were not heavy enough to inflict fractures. But a blow may have been sufficient to cause unconsciousness. Then, if she had been put in the bathtub with water, she drowned. Her lungs were wet with severe edema that, by itself, did not mean much without other abnormalities. Her heart and all other organs were absolutely healthy. I handled this case as homicide with numerous pictures of the body and microscopic study of the internal organs, sending to the toxicology lab blood and other samples for drugs, alcohol, and medication tests. To the serology lab, I sent her blood and rape kit and put a rush on the case.

Toxicology results were negative for everything. No semen was found on the vaginal, oral, or rectal swabs. From the police investigator, I received information that she had been found in a questionably secured apartment and that the last time she had been seen was on the previous Friday. Her family called her on Saturday, Sunday, and Monday, but to no avail. On Tuesday her father, together with the super of the building, opened the door and found her submerged in the bathtub. I talked with the father on the phone, and he told me that she had been a very healthy person. He said he had talked with her on Thursday, and she had told him she was supposed to work on Friday, Saturday, and Sunday. She did work on Friday, but she did not show up on Saturday. They called her, but nobody answered.

Her boyfriend called the father twice and told the parents he could not come to her funeral because two weeks prior he had been involved in a motor vehicle accident and had broken his leg. The father said he was sure that she had been killed. Her apartment key was missing, but the door was locked, yet her VCR and TV had disappeared. I passed this information on to the detective.

I certified the cause of death: drowning. Blunt force injury to head. Manner: Homicide.

I never was called to a grand jury or a trial. Probably, this case is still open. But the diagnosis leaves no doubt.

***

Another case of drowning in the bathtub differs from the first one by the medical history of the young woman and the findings. I had this case long ago, just after a couple of years with OCME, and this case definitely puzzled me. A young black woman in her early twenties was placed in a very respectable New York hospital with schizophrenia, a psychiatric disorder. She was taken to the hospital because she had dangerous thoughts toward herself and others. At the hospital, she received the medications Novane and Cogentine.

The hospital psychiatrist gave me the following information. The patient was found in the bathtub submerged in water. She did not have a history of seizures disorder that could be a cause of her incapacity in the water and drowning. The psychiatrist also denied the patient's suicidal attempts or thoughts. He said, "Yes, she was depressed because her newborn child was taken from her. The reason for that was a positive toxicology test for drugs in the child and mother. The patient was placed in a shelter, and the child was given to the grandmother. The woman was raised in a foster home and frequently ran away. She refused to take the Prozac that was prescribed to her."

Another psychiatrist gave me a little more information about the deceased. In the hospital, she was isolated and depressed, staying mostly in bed. She did not get along with her three roommates. And she had a history of a previous suicidal attempt. She was found at 3:45 pm face down in bathtub half-filled with water. She had been seen alive at 3:30 pm. A nurse and other staff pulled her out of the water, placed her on a bed, and started CPR. When the doctor arrived, she observed the nude body, which had a hardly palpable carotid pulse and fixed dilated pupils. The patient was transferred to the ICU where she remained for eighteen hours, developing respiratory distress, pulmonary edema, and multiple organ failure. She finally succumbed.

I performed the autopsy on this young female. She did not have any signs of trauma and no petechial hemorrhages. She had horizontal scar on the lower abdomen (from a C-section) and signs of hospital intervention: a tube in the mouth and multiple intravenous marks and lines. Her skull and brain were normal. Both lungs showed edema but no other abnormalities. Her heart was absolutely normal as well as all other organs. Initially, after the autopsy, I put the cause of death: pending further study. I had to check her blood and other fluids and organs for drugs and medication, study her organs under the microscope, and request the result of the police investigation.

The toxicology study was negative for drugs and medication. The microscopic study did not reveal anything unusual. The police report did not show anything suspicious, and her roommates were not involved in her drowning. So, I was facing the strange manner of her death: suicide. It was very difficult for me to imagine how she herself could do it, against the instinct to breathe that would cause all of us to pull our heads out of water. I experimented to see how long I could stay submerged, but I barely could do it for less than two minutes. So how could she? I went to the chief medical examiner with all the materials to discuss the case. After the discussion our conclusion was—cause of death: anoxic encephalopathy (lack of oxygen to the brain) due to drowning. Manner: suicide. Why? Homicide was excluded by the police investigation. Other people were not involved in her drowning. It could not have been an accident because the bathtub with water was not a sea or a river. Our conclusion was based on her history of depression and her previous suicide attempt.

***

About ten years after this case, I had another case of young woman found dead in a bathtub filled with water. Of course, during these years I did have cases of old people or very sick people found dead in the bathtub, but these cases were different; the old people had cardiac diseases or stroke, or they were debilitated by tumors or other serious illnesses. This case was much more complicated.

A young black woman was found in a hot water bathtub by her girlfriend. The initial information that I received from our medical investigator was, "A twenty-one year old female, no past medical history, expired in a tub full of hot water. Scene investigation reveals the apartment to be without evidence to suggest a foul play. No illegal drugs, drug paraphernalia, nor weapons found. By report, the deceased was discovered to have expired by her roommate lying in a bathtub full of hot water this morning, possible drowning. No criminality or foul play." The police detective from our office also gave me information that he had received from a detective of the precinct who was on the scene (the usual chain of information): The deceased was found by the girlfriend in bathtub, unresponsive, and 911 was called. The girlfriend came with her boyfriend at night. They heard the running water but thought that their friend was taking a bath. They went to sleep on a couch. When they awakened, the water in bathroom was still running, and they broke the door with tools to gain the entry. The deceased was found submerged face up with foam coming from her nose. The girlfriend had key access to the apartment; she had last spoken to the deceased the day before. The girlfriend also found an empty bottle of gin in the living room. Steam and hot water were in the bathroom when she entered. The deceased was not depressed and did not have a psychiatric history. She did not use drugs. With this information, I received the case.

In front of me on the morgue table was a young black woman in her twenties, measuring five feet, four inches and weighing one hundred and eighty pounds. Rigidity was absent. Fixed libidity was present on the back. There was a slippage of skin at the front and back on the upper and lower extremities and also on the face—the right cheek and nose. From the picture at the scene of the investigation, I saw the foam coming from the mouth and nose. Foam is evidence that she was alive on the moment of submersion because it is produced by the mixture of air, mucus, and water in the presence of respiratory movement. She did not have any trauma. Both lungs were edematous (containing a lot of fluid), as we usually see in any cardiac death. The heart and other organs were normal. The stomach contained about twenty-five milliliters of brownish fluid.

Of course, I dealt with this case as a homicide. Thus, multiple pictures were taken overall. Submitted to the forensic labs were blood, fingernails, head hair, pubic hair, and swabs from the mouth, vagina, and anus. The brain was put in formalin for the study by a neuropathologist, and various small pieces of internal organs were sent to the histology lab for study under the microscope for possible diseases. Young adults may drown in the bathtub if they are under the influence of drugs or alcohol, and an empty bottle of gin had been present on the table of the deceased's apartment. So, the tests would be very indicative. Also, a police report of further investigation was requested.

The young woman's mother called me, and I talked with her couple of times. She sounded like a very intelligent woman, and she had two other younger children. She was devastated by death of her older daughter. She gave me information that her daughter had been a very healthy woman with no problems, without seizures disorder, drug usage, or suicidal attempts. She did use alcohol but was not "a drunkard." The mother did not suspect her daughter's friend in any criminal activity. I explained to her my plan of action and promised to speed up the investigation of the case.

The toxicology report showed absence of drugs but presence of alcohol in the blood and in the vitreous humor (the clear eyeball fluid). The level of alcohol was equal three to four drinks. It is generally agreed that the alcohol concentration in blood decreases by a drink every hour. Considering the information that the girlfriend had heard the running water long before she found her dead, and assuming that the young woman was taking bath, I could deduce that initially the alcohol level was much higher than the toxicology report showed. The girlfriend also stated that the deceased had a habit of sometimes sleeping in the bathtub with water. Many people do that when tired. Meanwhile, the brain and microscopic studies were normal. On my request, the police again and again interviewed the girlfriend and her boyfriend, excluding their involvement in the death. I received another report from the detective that completely excluded her friend in any criminal activity.

Based on my findings, I certified the cause of death as drowning. Manner: accidental. But my main boss reviewed the case and came to a different conclusion. The cause of death was changed to "cardiac arrhythmia of unknown etiology. Manner: natural."

The diagnosis of drowning is a diagnosis of exclusion, and many things have to be taken into consideration. Alcohol, drugs, diseases such as epilepsy, amyotrophic lateral sclerosis, berry aneurysm with rupture, and heart diseases must be excluded. In 1981, before I was in the field of forensic pathology, the boss wrote in his case sample, "But simple drunkenness usually does not cause rapid incapacitation, and its victim remain responsive to stimulation, such as facial submersion, for an appreciable interval before the onset of deep coma. Therefore, one does not drown in a bathtub unless he or she is ***unwilling or unable*** to raise the head."

I consulted the case with my former boss and teacher.

"If you ask five forensic pathologists their opinions, they will give you five different answers," was his response.

It is a difficult case, indeed.

SUDDEN INFANT DEATH

In 1985 I started my fellowship in forensic pathology at the Office of Chief Medical Examiner in Detroit. It was an active and a very busy office indeed, where I performed four hundred cases during my one year tenure as a fellow. Among those were a great number of the so-called Sudden Infant Death Syndrome (SIDS) cases, and that definitely amazed me. As a pathologist for thirteen years back in the Old World, I saw and performed a lot of pediatric death cases, but I never had seen SIDS—perhaps because these cases were directed to forensic pathologists. As a pediatrician, I also never had direct experience with the SIDS. But it so happened that shortly before my immigration, I had exposure to a good monograph by a Soviet forensic pathologist, Akopian, who described his study of a large group of SIDS deaths. He actually found in every case some contributory factors such as respiratory viral infection, diarrhea, or some other medical condition, which made me think that those cases were not so "sudden," especially considering the vulnerability of infants.

Now, working in forensic pathology, I immediately got involved in cases where infants were determined to be victims of sudden death, and SIDS was the most common cause of death for the age group from one to twelve months. One of the first such cases that I encountered was a two month old baby who was found in the crib face down on the stomach, as was the customary position for American infants. On autopsy I did not find anything that could explain this death. The investigation report from the detective (they usually investigate such cases) did not raise any suspicion either. My microscopic study did not reveal pneumonia or any other abnormality, for that matter. According to the definition, this was a typical case of SIDS by exclusion of all other causes. I went to our deputy to discuss the case and expressed my opinion of the cause of death. "I think that this baby suffocated being face down on his stomach," I said. "He could not raise his head to release the nose and mouth. Thus, I think that the cause of death is asphyxia."

"No, the babies face down on their stomachs still could turn their faces aside, as many studies of the respectable American pediatric pathologists showed. You have to read these articles," he said.

I tried to explain to him that back in the USSR it was a custom to put all infants on their backs. The infants were tightly wrapped in the cotton diapers (at that time, we did not have disposable diapers), their arms wrapped along the torso and legs. The head would be facing up and free. This kind of "diapering" preserved the horizontal position of the child face up, and thus excluded possibility of suffocation due to being face down into a pillow or a soft mattress. In fact, our infants were diapered as Egyptian mummies to preserve their position. I raised my two sons the way my mother, our grandmothers, and great-grandmothers had raised their children—by restricting all movements of the infants by this kind of diapering when they were not awake. When the infants *were awake,* from the age of two months, sometimes even earlier, and under a parent's supervision, the child could be put on its stomach on a firm surface, and the little baby would struggle to raise its heavy head with its weak and unstable neck. It was like an exercise. Only after four to six months, depending how strong the baby was, would we release the hands from the "mummy" position of diapering and allow lying on the stomach with the nose turned aside. Our children were not free according to the American standard, but this was an ancient tradition that protected infants from suffocation.

My second case looked even more bizarre to me in

interpretation of the infant death as "sudden" because the grieving parents were two very handsome black people. They were strong and tall, and they put their baby between them in their bed. The autopsy, the following investigation, and a study of the case did not reveal anything.

"I think that they—of course, not intentionally—suffocated him by overlying!" I insisted in my discussion of the case.

I was told, "No, it is the custom in this country to put baby in the bed with the parents, if they wish."

Apparently, I was from Mars, so I started to read articles, keeping my mouth shut as a resident who was here to learn and not to teach, especially in this country with such advanced medicine.

There were numerous articles describing SIDS, also called "crib death," coming from renowned schools, describing incidences and problems of identification of infants at risk, characteristics of affected infants, numerous epidemiologic factors, and multiple hypotheses. Infection, especially viral infection, according to the authors, could well serve as the "trigger mechanism" in the infant at risk. Infant botulism was mentioned as the cause for a small group of SIDS victims. DPT (Diphteria, Pertussis, and Tetanus) immunization was suspected in twelve infants after their inoculation in Tennessee, but then intensive investigation determined that the death rate did not exceed the number that might have been expected in that population. Psychological effects of sudden infant death syndrome on surviving family members were discussed, and role of government in current research was emphasized. These all were very respectable, if not convincing, and I, as a fellow, stopped venturing my personal opinion.

Upon completion of my fellowship in Detroit, I joined the OCME in New York City, the big office with big laboratories and services. There I found a new special SIDS program headed by a PhD in social studies, an intelligent and smart woman. Of course, the number of autopsies was also much higher than in Detroit, and among those we had a lot of cases labeled as

SIDS—the well established diagnosis among pediatricians and forensic pathologists, well known to parents "who had no power to predict or prevent this mysterious disease." Every case of child sudden death at home that we received to the office had a detective report, and if the case did not raise suspicion and we did not find any trauma from the x-ray or during the autopsy, and if the microscopic study of all internal organs was negative, then we called the case SIDS.

I was actually amazed by the prevalence of SIDS in New York at that time. In each and every case, the diligent SIDS program leader PhD would write a compassionate letter to the parents, and not once but twice—the first time after the autopsy, explaining to the parents what more would be done to study the cause of death, and the second time after finalizing the case with the diagnosis of SIDS. Obvious and suspicious was that the extremely high rate of SIDS appeared in the population of low socioeconomic status—in the families from economically disadvantaged communities, often when the mothers were drug abusers. In some cases, the children died while under care of babysitters who were not well qualified. I never had a case of SIDS from a family of high socioeconomic status. How was it possible? In some cases, the infants had a history of cold, running nose, and fever. True, I never found bronchitis or pneumonia in this group of infants, but I did observe the microscopic signs of laryngitis.

Not once did I express my opinion to my colleagues or to the SIDS program coordinator about it being wrong to put babies in the bed face down—that they were unable to turn the face aside with their weak necks, particularly if they had a pillow under the face or some kind of soft material, blanket, or mattress, which could asphyxiate the child. Also, if the child happened to have a cold with a stuffed or running nose, the position would additionally obstruct breathing, or the same might happen if she or he regurgitated food in a face down position on the stomach. Even worse might happen when the child slept between parents—the established custom in the society. It was so easy to accidentally overlay a baby, to shift a blanket onto a child's face, or for the adult to put a shoulder or arm on the little face and nose, causing asphyxia.

Meanwhile, multiple research articles, which cited each other, conferences, committees, and funds for SIDS study, continued to grow. We kept using these articles and research as a textbook. One of the articles by a respectable forensic pathologist considered the simultaneous sudden infant death syndrome in twins. Nine cases of twin infants who had suddenly and simultaneously died were described, two of which the author had examined personally. In his summary, the author emphasized that "in the past, the sudden death of the previously healthy infant at home was often attributed to the negligence of the parents. With increased understanding of the condition now termed SIDS, physicians recognize that lack of parental care is not the cause of this type of death."

In another editorial article of a medical journal, an author wrote that "from biblical times until recently, virtually all cases of sudden unexpected death in infants were indiscriminately ascribed to maternal overlying, either accidental or intentional. During the past century, it gradually became clear that overlying could not be a cause of all such infant deaths since death-scene investigations established that many infants were sleeping alone at the time of death. Now overlying as a cause is rarely diagnosed." The author continued, citing a veterinarian, "It is also relevant to note that overlying is the commonest cause of neonatal mortality in some mammalian species." But we of course are a little different, and he concluded that "sharing a bed with a young infant is the common and acceptable practice that has psychological benefits." His conclusion gave a green light to the wrong practice for infants!

Some years passed and eventually I started to observe signs of a different trend, one that made more sense to me. Even at the same year as the above mentioned editorial, an article by a not so famous pathologist appeared, who in his twenty-six cases, accompanied by good scene investigation, came to conclusion that there was strong circumstantial evidence of accidental death in six cases and various possible causes of death other than SIDS in the other cases, including accidental asphyxiation by an object in the crib, smothering by overlying while sharing the bed, hyperthermia, and even shaken baby syndrome. I remember discussing this article with one of the deputies. She ignored this study as not respectable.

In 1992 the American Academy of Pediatrics finally reversed the long-held conventional wisdom, recommending a new sleep position after the studies around the world had demonstrated an association between SIDS and the prone position. In Britain and New Zealand, research showed a 50 % drop in the SIDS rate when babies were put to bed on their backs. The American pediatricians began instructing parents to put their newborns to sleep on their backs rather than on their stomachs!

In 1995 I was a participant in the Forensic Pathologists' Conference in California, and I came across a presentation about simultaneous sudden death in twins. In there, there was big doubt about SIDS, and it was recommended to put the cause of death as "undetermined." From 1995, I had never put the diagnosis of SIDS in the cases that I had doubts about.

In the following years, the SIDS rate plummeted by 30 %. We definitely felt a diminishing of the SIDS cases. The PhD chief of the SIDS program left for another, probably more challenging, job, and her position was filled by a new person. The last time I heard a report, the amount of cases was remarkably small. Part of this, I think, is an improving quality of our studies, which eliminated the previously practiced indiscriminately standard approach to diagnostics of SIDS and better investigation of cases by well-prepared and trained medical investigators. An excellent book, *The Death of Innocents*, a true story of murder medicine and high-stakes science by Richard Firstman and Jamie Talan, published in 1997, showed that 5–10% of deaths attributed to SIDS are actually homicide. We no longer believe in repeated SIDS in one family. One unexplained infant death in a family might be SIDS, and only if we really did not find a good explanation after a very thorough investigation; two is very suspicious. Three is homicide. Nevertheless, even with the wider use of instructions from pediatricians concerning the right position of the child, teenage mothers in low income families continue to put their babies in the wrong position. The practice of sleeping with the babies is also not eliminated.

In the late 1990s, I received a one month old black female infant that was found by her older brother, age seventeen, who watched the child when the parents were at work. After feeding the baby, the brother put her on the couch, and about two hours later, he found the child unresponsive. On autopsy, the child had a slightly flat nose with whitish discoloration around it. There were no signs of trauma; x-ray, toxicology, and histology of the internal organs were normal. I certified the cause of death as undetermined. Manner: undetermined.

Over a year later, from the same family another female infant was found dead. This baby was premature, a twin, four days old. The mother went to store and left the premature twins and another nineteen month old child in the car with the same teenager who was now eighteen-plus. The windows of the car were slightly open according to the teenager. At home, one of twins became very pale, started to have difficulties with breathing and was hospitalized with a very high body temperature on admission. The child died, and I finalized the case as hyperthermia due to elevated environmental temperature; prematurity. Manner: accidental. This death was the second in the same family over a one-year span, and under no circumstances was I going to diagnose it as SIDS.

I remained very skeptical about SIDS as a diagnosis because it just shows that the child died suddenly, but does not show the cause of death, and it actually covers up negligence, and accidental, or even homicidal manner. The diagnosis "undetermined" with manner natural is another way to cover for such sudden death cases. The right pronouncement for such cases, I think, is the diagnosis undetermined with manner undetermined as an honest statement about our inability to determine the cause of death at the present time. The advancements in techniques and quality of medical examination in all specters of the death study including bacteriology, virology, and scrupulous investigation will undoubtedly provide more precise differentiation for the causes and manners of death for these sad cases.

MYSTERY OF THE TWELVE DAY OLD BABY

Once I received the case of a twelve day old white boy who was brought dead by his mother to the hospital clinic. All resuscitation attempts were unsuccessful. When I came to the autopsy room and looked at the body, I was shocked. The boy looked exactly like children and corpses in pictures from the Auschwitz or Buchenwald concentration camps—those shocking pictures we grew familiar with after World War II.

The body was twenty inches in length, normal for the age, but it weighed only nineteen hundred grams. His whole appearance was of a dehydrated and starving child with dry, thin skin that easily made wrinkles because of the absence of underlying fat. His sternum, ribs, and all other bony structures were prominent, covered by very thin, pale skin. His cheeks, usually round and puffy in newborns, were absolutely flat. The chief medical examiner, who routinely came to review the daily autopsies, was also in disbelief. What was it negligence? Child abuse?

The autopsy did not reveal any of the signs of trauma that we carefully exclude in a child's case, when we perform preliminary x-ray studies of the whole body. Multiple Kodachromes were taken. The autopsy showed that the child did not have any congenital abnormalities which could have caused such malnutrition and dehydration. Pieces of all internal organs were taken for the consequent microscopic study, as were the usual samples for the toxicology lab. The brain was saved in formalin for neuropathology tests by our specialist in this field. In addition, the blood was sent to the Health Department for a microbiology study. During the autopsy, I noticed that the child's stomach and his small and large intestines were absolutely empty. All organs weighed a little less than could be expected in such a cachexic, dehydrated child.

Because I did not find obvious cause of death, I made the initial diagnosis "pending further study." I had to study a lot of things. I did not know history of this child. I needed to talk with the parents, his doctors, the detective, and our medical investigators. I needed to see the slides of the internal organs under the microscope to exclude any disease, and I needed to review the results of reports from the toxicology and microbiology labs and the results of the brain study by our neuropathologist.

From our medical investigator, I received information that this was the first child of a thirty year old mother, who was a dancer. The father was a musician of age thirty-five. The mother had a normal prenatal course. The child's weight at birth was twenty seven hundred grams (5 lb 15 oz), and he was full term at birth. The child's Apgar score, which evaluates color, respiration, reflex response, and muscle tone was normal a 9/9. There were no observed gross physical abnormalities. The child had been active and alert with good muscle tone, and he had been fed by breast when he was discharged from the hospital two days after his birth. The family had a private pediatrician who had seen the child seven days prior to his death, and everything had been normal at that time, according to the pediatrician.

The doctor from the hospital that admitted the dead child noticed the "flat" reaction of his mother.

Two weeks after the autopsy, a doctor from another hospital, the chief of a genetic laboratory, called me, and we discussed the case. He told me that the mother's amniotic fluid had been tested for chromosomal abnormalities and none had been identified during the pregnancy. The midwife, who delivered the baby and had just heard about the baby's death, also came to my office to discuss the case. She repeated the basic information—that the baby had been delivered as normal with good weight and height and discharged from the hospital on the second day (the usual procedure). She said that the mother had never called her during the past twelve days. She called the mother herself, and the mother had told her that she had enough milk and fed the baby when the child wanted to be fed. According to the midwife, the mother was an articulate and intelligent person. The mother had called the family doctor three days before the child's death and told the doctor that the child's fontanel (the soft membrane between the incompletely ossified head bones of fetuses and infants) was flat and that the child had constipation. The doctor had not been concerned about either, and the mother had taken the baby to upstate New York. She had come back to New York City two days later. According to the mother, she had last fed the baby at night, and in the morning the child did not wake up. She thought that he was still sleeping. A neighbor, who came to the home, had noticed the strange condition of the child and told the mother, who called the doctor. The doctor had asked the mother to bring the child to his office immediately. She did, and the child had been sent to the hospital immediately. On admission, the baby was dead and had a low rectal temperature. The latter suggested that the child had already been dead for several hours.

The father called me and gave the following information: The baby had been fine three days before his death and had had normal bowel movements and urinated ten times per day. (How could he count that in a twelve day old baby?) But they had noticed he had a flat fontanel and called the pediatrician. The doctor had told them that it was "not sufficient" for worries, and they had taken the child to their place in upstate New York. The mother had had enough milk and was feeding the baby ten times a day, just "when the baby asked." For the last two days, the child had not had a bowel movement. The day before the child had been found unconscious, he had had red urine, and they thought about dehydration. They did not give the child water because "the doctor told them that the milk was enough." On Saturday, the child had been unconscious, and they had brought him to the doctor.

I called the family pediatrician and confirmed the story about the flat fontanel call. "How come this call did not warn you about the condition of the child?" I asked the pediatrician.

"I am receiving too many calls about flat or budging fontanels from parents and usually do not worry about it. And you are not a pediatrician, you are a pathologist, a forensic pathologist, in fact, and it is not your area of expertise," the pediatrician quite arrogantly finished, hanging up the telephone.

It was not exactly true because, with my background, I was a pediatrician by education. I had graduated from medical school with the pediatric subspecialty in the former USSR. And I had worked as a pediatrician for the first four years after graduation. Of course, it was not the area of my expertise now, but what I had learned in medical school and from my short pediatric practice was that the infant must ALWAYS be seen and carefully followed by the pediatrician when a complaint arises, because the infant may develop unexpected threatening situations very quickly. If I had been this pediatrician, I would have asked the mother to bring the child to me immediately.

The toxicology results were negative for drugs and medication, but the vitreous humor (fluid from the eyes) showed severe dehydration. The brain study by our neuropathologist did not reveal anything abnormal. No organisms were isolated in the child's blood, according to the report from the Department of Health. The microscopic study of all internal organs showed the atrophy of muscles. That could have resulted from malnutrition or a congenital muscular disorder.

It did not look to me that the child had been fed normally. Had the mother had enough milk? Had the child been able to suck her breast milk? According to the parents, she had had milk, and the child had received it ten times a day. But as I mentioned, the stomach and bowels were completely empty. I asked the detective to bring in the child's used diapers. They were brought together with the absolutely clean unused diapers. I was pleasantly surprised to see the unused beautiful cotton brand diapers with initials (not standard paper diapers, as most people nowadays are using). But the used soiled diapers had a very small barely seen stool smudging. It did not appear to me at all that the baby had eaten and had normal bowel movements.

The case was complicated, and I went to consult it with the chief of pediatric pathology of NYU. She analyzed everything very carefully. The case was also consulted with the neuropathologist of the same university. As I already mentioned, the child's muscles showed atrophy that could have resulted from starvation or a congenital abnormality (floppy infant?). But there was no family history, and the child had been normal at birth without any neuromuscular abnormality. The parents themselves did not give any history of the floppy child. Floppy child, or hypotonic infant, is a very rare inherited condition with weakness of skeletal muscles and the possibility of a failure to thrive. But it would be difficult to diagnose such a condition in this twelve day old baby.

I did not have any information about the maternal postpartum depression that could be the origin of child neglect.

Finally I went with everything to discuss the case with my boss, the chief medical examiner, in the presence of the first deputy. They both agreed with my diagnosis of "malnutrition and dehydration," but were in doubt about "of unknown etiology."

"Could it be negligence?" they both were asking. That would have changed the forensic pathologist's definition of the manner of death to "homicide." It was true that the parents did not seek immediate medical attention. But I was quite persistent, because I thought that the baby was a wanted first child in this professional family. His soft cotton brand diapers with the initials suggested to me the parents' love and thoughtfulness. The mother had called the doctor with her concern about the baby. It was not clear if the child had some kind of congenital disease that we, with all our resources, could only suspect but not confirm. I did not feel that a finding of homicide was undoubtedly justified to open this family to the social workers' and family court investigators' sanctions and decisions. They could not do more than I had already done. And the parents were suffering enough. So, I insisted and put the cause of death: malnutrition and dehydration of unknown etiology. Manner of death: undetermined.

A week after my amendment of the death certificate, I was discussing the case with the child's mother. I explained that her child died of malnutrition and dehydration. She kept insisting that all these days the child had been sucking well and that she had had enough milk. The baby had not have diarrhea or vomiting and had never been sick, having only constipation, she said. I continued explaining that she could not insist on good feeding as she had never checked before the feeding and after it if to see if she really had enough milk and if the child had received it. I also explained to her that I had consulted the case with very experienced specialists and the congenital abnormality could not be excluded. The mother told me that she was not aware of anybody in her or her husband's family who had a congenital abnormality. I recommended that she have herself and her husband checked by a gynecologist and a genetic specialist. She persisted, so I told her that I could not understand how she and her husband did not notice that the child was loosing weight dramatically and seek medical attention immediately—such malnutrition and dehydration had not developed overnight. She told me that they did not realize how serious it was because the child had been active and sucking well all those days.

I was very surprised when, after couple of weeks, my boss, the chief medical examiner of New York, called me to his office, frowning angrily, and read a letter from the family's lawyer, accusing me of a tough investigation that terrorized the family. I could not believe it!

"It is ironic! I was the only in our office who insisted on the undetermined manner and against negligence," I exclaimed.

My boss, who supervised and consulted many cases, may

have not remembered right away the essence of this case, reading the lawyer's letter and becoming angered with me, but after I reminded him of the case, he softened. "I will write them a letter," was his response.

I have not heard from the family or their lawyer again.

HANGING BY PACIFIER

Never before in my practice as a forensic pathologist had I had a case of a child who hanged himself by the pacifier. As all other people, I considered a pacifier to be a harmless device to soothe and quiet a crying baby. Not any more. This ten month old, well-developed black boy was found unresponsive, lifeless, hanging from the crib by a pacifier string. He was immediately brought to the hospital, where he was pronounced dead on arrival. The horizontal ligature mark was present on his neck.

I performed an autopsy on the body of the ten months child. He had a normal height and weight, and there were no signs of trauma of the skull or other parts of the body, except for the two millimeter wide pale ligature mark with reddish margins. The marks were horizontal at the front, oblique on the right side of the neck, horizontal on the left side, and they turned vertically at the middle of the back. There were some signs of medical intervention by hospital personnel, mostly resuscitation marks. An x-ray was performed before I started the autopsy, and the child's body was photographed. All organs were normal. Blood, bile, and small pieces of internal organs were taken for toxicology tests. Small pieces of internal organs were taken for the histology lab. A police report was requested.

The cause of the child's death was clear: asphyxia due to hanging by the pacifier cord. The manner was not yet clear because I needed the detailed police investigation report. The police report came promptly. Information that I received said that the child was under care of the foster mother, who had other foster children in the house. This baby had been placed in the rear bedroom because the foster mother had a vacuum cleaner demonstration and did not want to bother the child with the noise. The foster mother's daughter went to check on the baby twenty to thirty minutes after he was left in the crib, and she had discovered him lifeless, unconscious, and hanging on the cord (shoe lace) from the crib. Everybody became frantic. The daughter's boyfriend immediately started CPR. The foster mother called the police and ran to emergency room of a nearby hospital to solicit help, but the result was negative. Then she ran home where the police had already arrived and called EMS. Upon arrival, the EMS immediately started resuscitation and took the child to the hospital. Nothing helped, and the child was pronounced dead on arrival.

There were other foster children in the house, all healthy and well fed. The foster mother had taken care of them during seven years, and she had had this boy from the time he was four and half months old. This was the first time that such a disaster had happened. The foster mother was devastated and visibly upset. The police investigator felt that it was an accident. All my other studies, histology and toxicology, were negative, and I certified the case as accidental.

In the late 1990s, I had a case of eight month old child who died because of asphyxia (suffocation) as a result of hanging. The child was trapped between the mattress and side of the crib. Strangulation in childhood is not a new issue. It has been studied for years and years, and is the subject of preventive regulations issued by the Consumer Product Safety Commission. High chairs, playpen mesh, pacifier cords, clothing—all may be objects causing strangulation. More information and targeted education are very important for prevention.

During my years as a medical examiner, I saw a lot of accidental deaths of children that could have been prevented. They are all in my memory, and very often I offer unsolicited advice to my daughters-in-law, who are raising my grandchildren.

"Do not leave your eight month old baby girl with the three year old brother in a bathtub with water," I say, and I immediately mention the example of the child drowning. Or I say, "Do not leave them alone playing outside on the street."

"But I am frequently watching them from the window," my daughter-in-law responds.

"Well, please go outside then. Stay there, and watch the kids."

My daughters-in-law get annoyed. They want to raise their kids independently and not be overly protective.

I say, "When you are exiting the elevator, do not allow the small child to leave or enter without your holding the child by the hand. Be careful with the child inside the elevator."

I had a case when an overweight mother, holding a lot of bags in her hands, tripped and fell on a child while exiting an elevator, causing the child's death due to skull fractures. And I am not at all sure that all these photo-elements in the elevators' doors are always sensitive to the height of a child. I give such advice in the elevator in our building to many nannies with children, and in response I often receive a nasty stare, or worse, the retort, "It is none of your business."

I worry when I see a tall father holding his beloved child on his shoulder and walking the streets of New York City. I mentally measure the distance between the child's head and the canopy that is overhanging the sidewalk or a tree branch that is protruding from the other side. It could hurt the child. And it does sometimes—I see it happen with the thin tree branch, but luckily it does not hurt the child badly. I outrun the father and give him a "look." At least, I get the small gratification that I am not paranoid.

CHILDREN WITH CONGENITAL ABNORMALITIES

Heart Abnormality

Mommy, I am dying!

A four year old girl is on the morgue table. She does not look dead. She looks as if she is sleeping. It is always very painful for me to perform autopsies of children despite my many years of experience. I feel the pain of the parents, and I take it personally, thinking of my children.

I received related information from the medical investigator that the girl collapsed while playing in the park. A short statement from the hospital said that the previously well child had been presented to a hospital as suddenly ill, vomiting, and fainting. She was then transferred to another hospital where, initially awake and alert, her functions soon became de-compensated. Her ECG became abnormal, and she developed cardiac arrest. In spite of maximal supportive care and prolonged resuscitative efforts, she went into irreversible shock leading to cardiopulmonary arrest.

As usual each morning, my boss, followed by a tall blonde female, a medical investigator, approached my table. My boss is a man of fifty-seven to fifty-eight, who has been trimmed by vigorous, daily one-hour morning exercise and a strict diet. He has an intelligent face, a slightly asymmetrical nose, and a voice that makes him sound older than he actually is. He is an author of many professional papers and books, and he is our "God" when it comes to complicated cases.

The boss's escort is a young, good-looking woman in her late twenties or early thirties, a former nurse and a recent addition to our staff, a smart woman who produces clearly written and complete investigation reports. I like her, and my boss's obvious fascination with her does not irritate me. They look good together, tall and lean, every morning descending from the first floor to the morgue in the basement, having small talk, joking, and looking pleased with each other. They usually proceed from table to table, apparently feeling superiority from being in charge. Probably it stimulates both of them. The boss is, I presume, the author of this good idea, described in the OCME orientation notes for new pathologists, "Never go home without dictating your autopsies; if you get hit by a bus, it is too bad; if you get hit by a bus leaving incomplete autopsies, it is a tragedy!"

"What is your thinking about the possible cause of death?" the boss asks me.

"It might be a congenital heart abnormality," I say, and he nods his agreement.

But of course, the first thing to exclude is a child's trauma. On the external examination there is nothing suspicious. There are not any external bruises, but this does not mean absence of bruises when the body is open. I carefully look at the x-ray films that we obtained prior to the autopsy. There are no fractures. We photograph the child's body at the front and the back.

The autopsy does not show anything wrong with the organs except the heart with its blood vessels. It quickly becomes obvious that the child indeed has a congenital heart abnormality. The child's left coronary artery originates from the same sinus as the right one, and that is wrong for a normal heart. The openings of both arteries are divided by a slight bridge of tissue. After its origin from the wrong place, the left artery proceeds by encircling the pulmonary artery that appears between this artery and the aorta. The right coronary artery, immediately after its origin, is smaller and shorter than usual. The left circumflex artery is unusually delicate, and the consequent microscopic study reveals fibroblastic proliferation (connective tissue growth). It is again abnormal because it narrows the internal space of the artery and diminishes blood supply to the heart.

The child's heart shows acute myocardial infarct with pale and reddish areas of the anterior and lateral walls of the left ventricle. There is also an old myocardial infarct with scarring of the posterior wall of the left ventricle. The entire heart looks like the heart of an old person with atherosclerotic cardiovascular disease. Of course, the infarcts were not caused by atherosclerosis; the child's coronary arteries are young. It is the wrong congenital origin of the left coronary artery, which became squeezed between the pulmonary artery, and the aorta that caused insufficient blood supply to the cardiac muscles, particularly during the child's activity, such as running. It is a very serious defect, and it is further complicated by the other congenital abnormality of the two blood vessels, right and circumflex, which prevented the heart from any compensation for the left coronary artery problem. In old people the gradual worsening of the coronary blood vessels gives them time to develop some opening of the small collateral blood vessels, thus diminishing the negative effect of the aging blood vessels. The child did not have such an opportunity.

After the autopsy, I received a call from one of the oldest pediatric cardiologists of the hospital where the child expired. He told me that the child's heart enzymes were elevated—that being consistent with my findings. The doctor reviewed the child's ECG which showed the recent and the old myocardial infarcts. He also told me that a month ago, according to the mother, the child complained of the chest pain. But who would take this complaint seriously from a four-year-old? On the last admission at the hospital, this four year old girl told her mother in the presence of the doctors, "Mommy, I am dying." Unfortunately, the poor girl was right.

The pediatric cardiologist recommended consulting the case with the chief of the pathology department, "a hell of a good cardio-pathologist." I showed the case to several good cardio-pathologists. At first, it was our first deputy, a very nice person to deal with. She ordered more microscopic slides of the heart and its blood vessels, implemented with the special stain. I rushed' the case through the labs because cases of the children, I think, must be finished as soon as possible. The death of the child is a huge tragedy for the parents—we must give the explanation as soon as possible. And I also went and discussed the case with the recommended chief of the pathology department, the editor of the cardiology journal. We all came to the final cause of death: "ischemic heart disease due to congenital blood vessels abnormality." It would be very difficult, if not impossible, for doctors to have arrived at this diagnosis on her admission to the hospital.

There was a very sad discussion with the child's mother to whom I explained the cause of death in detail.

***

I had just finished describing this case of the child's death due to abnormality of the coronary arteries, and on CNN.com/health, I stumbled on an article updated only two hours prior. The article "Doctors Report Rare Heart Attacks in Kids" (October 1, 2007) described a heart attack in a thirteen year old teenager and gave a reference to a report from Ohio documenting nine cases in kids as young as twelve, collected over the course of eleven years. I was glad to see that this information appeared publicly to make parents more alert to consult a doctor any time a child shows sudden chest pain. There could be many causes for the chest pain, including heart spasm, infection, muscle strain, stress or, as in the case described above, structural abnormalities.

Urinary Abnormality

Marco was a fifteen month old Hispanic child, the first and only child in the family. His dark brown eyes looked lovely on his slightly pale face, and his dark, straight hair was never trimmed, waiting for his third birthday. He smiled as his father, broadly and kindly. Marco was a beautiful child loved by his parents, by all neighbors in this tall, red brick project building in the Bronx, and by his Dominican grandparents whom Marco had visited just three months earlier. Marco's parents were very proud of him because Marco had taken the five-hour back and forth flights as a real macho boy—he did not cry. He drank his milk and ate his Farina wheat cereal. Recently he had started to talk, and when he had not had enough words, his facial expressions and hand movements had helped him express himself. Marco's parents, as all the other parents in the world, had not needed words to understand their lovely little boy.

Marco was born in the United States, not in the Dominican Republic as were his parents, and that meant that one day he might have been elected as the President of this country. His father dreamt about his bright future, and as the first step to that, he chose one of the best Manhattan hospitals as the place for his son's birth. The proud parents kept their appointments with the pediatrician every month. The child had been healthy, gaining weight, and developing well, according to the doctors who followed standards for children's development. Only once, had Marco had a gastrointestinal infection (diarrhea). A few months before, his parents had noticed that their child was "pushing hard to make urine," and they had immediately voiced their concern to the pediatrician.

Marco was examined by the pediatrician and referred to a pediatric urologist at the same facility, and the parents were informed that the child did not have any serious problems, that he was fine. Instructions were given to the parents on how to retract the foreskin of the penis in case of difficulties. The last time

Marco was seen by his pediatrician during a regular examination had been just one month prior, before the child became seriously ill. At that time, he had been alert and playful. His blood test had been normal, but a urine test had not been done.

In the middle of February, Marco fell ill. For three to four days, he had a cough, intermittent fever, and a decreasing appetite. His mother had given him Pedialyte and PediSure for two to three days. In the early morning, when Marco's father left home for work one day, the child still did not look too bad. Then, at 10:00 am, his wife called and said that Marco was crying and did not look well at all. The father immediately made an appointment with the pediatrician for 1:00 pm. At eleven o'clock his wife called him again, and then again after about an hour, this time to say that Marco was "crying harder." The worried father heard Marco crying very loudly in the background.

"He does not look well. He is pale, and his fingers and lips look blue," the mother told him.

"Go immediately to the hospital across the street."

His wife, who did not speak English, called a cousin who lived nearby and they walked together, with the child in their arms, to the nearest facility, the DTC clinic. They approached the registration area. The registered nurse of the clinic later told the detective that the mother entered the building hysterically crying "My baby, my baby."

The mother and the cousin had a concern, as the father later told me, that the staff at the clinic did not respond quickly and did not have any oxygen available. But according to the attending pediatrician, who was promptly summoned to the registration area, the child was pale, was not breathing, had no pulse, and was in a mild rigor. Oxygen was given—the child was intubated (the tube was inserted into the larynx through the mouth), and ACLS (resuscitation) protocols were administered. All attempts at resuscitation were unsuccessful. His rectal temperature became low. His condition was getting worse and worse. An IV line was attempted to the right leg. The quick blood test revealed an increase of the white blood cell count, while hemoglobin and spinal fluid remained normal. The blood was sent for culture, and the hospital even managed to make a skeletal series; however, it was not interpreted at that time. The x-ray results looked "like diffused pneumonia." All fluids were sent for culture and chemistry tests. The preliminary finding of the blood culture was positive for G negative bacilli E.Coli. Marco arrived to the clinic at 12:15 pm. He was pronounced dead at 12:34 pm.

The cause of death was unknown, and the child's body was referred to the Office of Medical Examiner for an autopsy. Both the parents and the hospital requested an autopsy.

On autopsy I did not see any sign of trauma. All his organs were normal, except the genitourinary tract. I was really very surprised to see severe changes in the genitourinary tract, the kidneys, ureters, and urinary bladder. His right kidney was markedly enlarged with multiple cysts filled with pus. His left kidney was also enlarged, but not so markedly, and its cysts had no pus. The ureters, the long narrow ducts that convey urine from the kidneys to the urinary bladder, were markedly distended. The urinary bladder was significantly distended and thick. I took small pieces of all internal organs for microscopic study. Blood was taken for microbiology and virology tests. As always, blood and urine were submitted for toxicology, and multiple photos were taken.

Temporary, I put the cause of death as "pending further study," because I wanted to study everything under the microscope and to have the results of the blood culture. I already knew the results of the hospital blood study, which revealed E. Coli. It was considered as more reliable than my postmortem blood culture test, which had more chances to be contaminated.

Microscopy of the internal organs proved what actually was seen already during the autopsy, the severe hypertrophy (significantly enlarged muscles) of the urine bladder—an indication that something made the urine bladder work harder than normal. Inflammation was also present. Both kidneys showed acute chronic pyelonephritis, and there was inflammation of both the kidneys and the pelvis. The blood culture results confirmed the hospital findings: E. Coli.

With all my results I went to the very good pediatric pathologist of New York University, with whom I had previously consulted some complicated cases. She was an intelligent, modest, small-framed lady in her fifties. Her accent showed her South American origin. I liked to discuss cases with her and appreciated her honest admission that not everything could be explained. We both agreed that the child had some congenital abnormality, but the precise nature of it was difficult to identify since the changes in the urinary tract had become severe. One possibility was the vesicolouretral reflux of urine from the bladder that most often occurs because of congenital malformation of the ureters. It is abnormal and predisposes the urinary tract to damage by bacterial infection. Because of that, the urine bladder and ureters are pushed to work harder than normal. The evidence of this condition was the markedly increased thickness of the urine bladder and ureters. It eventually was complicated by infection—acute and chronic pyelonephritis (infection of kidney)—and finally caused sepsis (blood infection) by E. Coli, the most common infection of the genitourinary tract.

I finalized the cause of Marco's death as E. Coli sepsis and uremia (insufficiency of kidney function) due to acute and chronic pyelonephritis and obstructive uropathy due to probable congenital urinary abnormality.

Urinary tract infections are the most common genitourinary disease of childhood. The symptoms and signs vary with age. Infants under two with urinary tract infections usually have non-urinary manifestations: feeding problems, failure to thrive, diarrhea, and unexplained fever. The disease can often masquerade as gastrointestinal illness, such as "colic," causing irritability and screaming periods. Marco did have a history of gastroenteritis (diarrhea) but only once, according his mother. By the way, she brought with her from the Dominican Republic amoxicillin, but she said she did not give it to the child.

So, how long did the child have this disease—months, weeks? Was it detectable and treatable? Yes, if urine studies followed by an evaluation of the urinary tract had been performed in a timely manner, treatment with antibiotics could have saved this child. Unfortunately, Marco did not show hardly any symptoms of his problem.

I called the father and explained the cause of Marco's death. I contacted the hospital, gave them the autopsy findings, and discussed the case. They wanted to see the parents and talk with them.

ONE OF FIVE COMMONLY
MISDIAGNOSED DISEASES

Eric, a twenty-three year old Hispanic man, was a newlywed who lived with his wife in a rented apartment. According to his family, he had started to complain of chest pain three days before he went to see about it. The pain became so severe that he went to emergency room of the nearby hospital. On an x-ray, he showed mild cardiomegaly (enlarged heart). His cardiac rate was fifty-eight, and his ECG was normal. He was seen by a doctor who prescribed a non-steroid analgesic, and he was sent home.

Over the next three days, he kept complaining of increasing chest pain, and at 8:00 pm of the third day, Eric collapsed and became unresponsive. The family called EMS; they administered resuscitation and transported him to the hospital. On arrival he was in cardiac arrest, unresponsive, without any vital signs. Examination in the hospital showed no trauma. They attempted resuscitation but were unsuccessful, and soon Eric was pronounced dead. The family denied any use of alcohol or drugs. There were no radiographic, serology, or toxicology studies performed.

The autopsy immediately revealed dissection of the ascending aorta with a rupture at two centimeters above the aortic valve, resulting in tamponade of the pericardial sac (that is, blood in the space between heart and capsule surrounding the heart). The heart of the deceased was markedly enlarged. The toxicology study for drugs and medication was negative. The microscopic study of the heart showed hypertrophy of the cardiac muscle; all other organs were normal.

I issued the cause of death: "dissecting thoracic aorta with heart tamponade due to hypertensive cardiovascular disease."

I requested and reviewed materials of the deceased's initial admission into the hospital three days before his death. He had complained of chest pain with radiation to the jaw. His chest x-ray showed some enlargement of the cardiac silhouette—mild cardiac cardiomegaly. And he had a history of hypertension, though it was never treated. Even on admission the patient had high blood pressure measured at 160/85. The diagnosis made was "musculoskeletal chest pain." He was released from the hospital. I am a pathologist, and cardiology is not an area of my expertise, but I think that patient's history of hypertensive disease should have been a red light to cause the doctors to treat him differently than just for "musculoskeletal chest pain."

Aortic dissection is highly lethal. In spite of the dramatic advances in its management, it is still a lethal disease. It is one of five commonly misdiagnosed diseases. In most cases, excruciating pain is the very first symptom. Although aortic aneurysm is primarily a disease of older people, the younger (less than age fifty-one) patients may also, but infrequently, have it. Once diagnosed, the patients may require surgery. Aneurismal disease presenting in the young adult is more likely to be symptomatic of and associated with more proximal aortic involvement than aneurismal disease in older patients. This group of patients is more at risk for early and aggressive aneurismal disease.

Eric should have been hospitalized immediately and carefully watched. A more thorough examination was needed to prompt surgery. Unfortunately, the latter has very high mortality rate as well. It was a big mistake to send him home with an analgesic. Young men of twenty-three do not come often to the emergency room just with "musculoskeletal pain." Of course, I reported the case to patient management. I just hope that this case was discussed at the hospital mortality conference and that the mistakes were found, at least retrospectively.

I would like to finish this sad case with a more optimistic

story. Going to an evening dance class, I ran onto a shabby man in his late forties whom I knew from a previous dance class. I was glad to see him because his overweight appearance with a protruded abdomen was always a big encouragement to me to take these classes. If he could do it, why couldn't I? I expressed my true excitement at seeing him again, and in response, he told me about his serious health problem that was happily resolved. He had a dissection of the thoracic aorta that was diagnosed and corrected surgically, and now he was dancing again. He was a lucky man to have excellent doctors who managed his case.

***

Hypertension, elevation of systolic and/or diastolic blood pressure, can be the primary disease or a secondary effect associated with other diseases, some of them potentially curable. I would like to describe one case that connects adrenal tumors and hypertension.

A thirty-two year old female with a history of hypertension disease expired in the hospital emergency room. She had been transported from home with shortness of breath that deteriorated rapidly to respiratory distress with pink frothy sputum coming from the nose and mouth. The drug test was negative. She was placed on ventilator support. The patient's clinical condition worsened with acute renal failure, of which the etiology remained unknown at that time.

The mother requested an autopsy. Our Office of Medical Examiner received the case, as the hospitals would usually send the family-requested cases to us. I never understood why this was necessarily so. In this case, the autopsy could have been done in the hospital in the presence of the clinical doctors—always a good teaching experience. But I stopped wondering about it a long time ago because the hospital doctors used to tell me that the families preferred to have the Medical Examiner Office on the case. Well, it was a big honor and trust for our office, and after such a statement, we definitely performed the autopsies. Pitifully, the clinical doctors were rarely present.

Before starting the autopsy, I received a telephone call from the mother of the deceased. She repeated the information about her daughter's hypertensive disease, without any special details, and insisted on checking her daughter for poisoning, without naming a particular suspect. We get such requests from families quite often as they have understandable difficulties in dealing with the deaths of their loved ones.

I performed the autopsy on the black female who appeared consistent with the stated age of thirty-two and was of normal height, but overweight. Her lungs showed severe edema and congestion. Her heart was enlarged with left ventricular hypertrophy, and that was consistent with her history of hypertensive cardiovascular disease. Her coronary arteries had a mild degree of atherosclerosis, as usual at this age. The liver and spleen were normal, and her kidneys had a granular surface that was also consistent with the hypertensive disease. The important finding was that the left adrenal had a well encapsulated tumor, eleven by eight by four centimeters in size, which grossly looked like pheochromocytoma with its soft appearance and yellowish-white to reddish-brown color on the cut section. But of course, microscopic and toxicology studies were in order. For the time being, I put as a cause of death as "pending further study," and I called the mother of the deceased with my preliminary findings and explanations of the further steps.

After couple of weeks, I had everything in place to finalize the cause of death. Her toxicology result was negative for drugs and medication except for the medication that she received in the hospital. The tumor, as I suspected, was pheochromocytoma.

Pheochromocytoma is a tumor of chromaffin cells which secrete catecholamine hormone and cause hypertension. In about 80% of the cases, they are found in the adrenal glands. They appear with equal frequency in both sexes and are usually benign in 95% of the cases. The most prominent feature is hypertension which may be paroxysmal or persistent and is rarely absent. There are many other symptoms that could raise suspicion for pheochromocytoma as a cause of hypertension, and among them are rapid pulse, sweating, postural hypotension (change of blood pressure with the change of body position), rapid breathing, flushing, cold and clammy skin, and a sense of impending doom. All these symptoms, of course, could be present in other conditions and diseases.

Pheochromocytoma is a rare and usually curable cause of hypotension. Pregnancy can elicit clinical manifestation of the otherwise unrecognizable tumor. The diagnosis of pheochromocytoma is made when free metaphrines and/or the presence of certain urinary products are found in the blood plasma. But these blood and urine tests are not part of routine procedures. They must be particularly ordered when the diagnosis is suspected. Then, the treatment of choice is surgical removal of the tumor.

Unfortunately the diagnosis was not suspected; the tumor was not removed, and the young woman died.

SPONTANEOUS CORONARY ARTERY DISSECTION

A thirty-three year old woman, working in her home kitchen, called her husband complaining of not feeling well. When he arrived, she was unconscious. EMS was immediately called. They started resuscitation with defibrillation, and they delivered her to a hospital in the state of cardiac arrest, with no pulse and blood pressure, and with fixed and dilated eyes. One hour after admission, in spite of all efforts, she was pronounced dead. Seven weeks earlier, this woman had delivered a baby by C-section without any further complications. She did not have any medical problems before or during the pregnancy. The hospital tentative diagnosis was: "Probably, pulmonary embolism. Disseminated intravascular coagulation?"

The hospital pathologist referred this case to the Office of Medical Examiner because the young woman had died in a very short period of time, and the cause of her death was unclear. The doctor might have also thought about drugs as a cause of her death. We, at OCME, had an excellent toxicology laboratory where multiple varieties of typical and atypical drugs and medication could be studied.

On autopsy I saw a well-developed Hispanic woman with the middle abdominal scar from a Cesarean section. Marks of resuscitation on the chest, tubes in the mouth and nose, and multiple intravenous lines were all signs of the hospital intervention. She did not have scars left by chronic intravenous narcotism. Then, I performed the internal examination and studied all her organs. Her heart had a normal weight, and two coronary arteries, the left descending and the right posterior, were normal. But even on gross examination I noticed a horizontal dark red discoloration along the distribution of the left circumflex artery. Further sectioning of this blood vessel showed that it was completely occluded by the dark red thrombus-blood clots. The occlusion started right at the origin of the artery and extended to its end.

All other organs were completely normal.

It was 1987, and at that time I was courageous enough to put the cause of death immediately as I initially deduced it; after all, we could always use the opportunity to amend the case if something new transpired in the post-autopsy studies. Some years later, we all started to be more cautious, preferring preliminary "pending further study" on about every second case. Now I think it is a wise decision to complete the entire study first and only then put the final diagnosis, avoiding unnecessary mistakes or amendments. In either case, though, the revealed truth would not be obstructed.

Again, for this case I put the cause of death right after the autopsy as "acute thrombosis of the left circumflex coronary artery." Atherosclerotic coronary artery disease, complicated by acute thrombosis, was the usual cause of sudden death in older people. But it was quite unusual in a young person.

To my big surprise, when I received microscopic slides of the heart and the left circumflex coronary artery that looked like thrombosis (blood clots) at autopsy, I discovered the rare pathology of the coronary artery—*dissection of the coronary artery.* This rare condition occurs sometimes in pregnant or post delivery women, the cause of which remains unknown in spite of some theories about it. I had never had such case before, but it definitely taught me to look more carefully at so called thrombus of the coronary arteries and not to rely on their gross appearance only. Histology of the coronary arteries must be performed, and it might show that these cases are more frequent than we thought.

In fact, being alert for this diagnosis after that case, I diagnosed another two occurrences: one of them a forty-six year old woman and the other a forty year old man. Both had sudden death. The woman did not have hypertensive cardiovascular disease, was neither pregnant nor had recently delivered a baby, and the man did not have any medical history at all.

Recently, I have read in a newspaper that one experienced pathologist was in big trouble after missing such diagnosis as a cause of death of a young woman, giving the wrong diagnosis of homicidal death instead. This rare diagnosis must be on our differential list of sudden deaths.

PRIMARY CARDIAC TUMOR

A healthy twenty-nine year old Hispanic woman started to choke at night, "by air" as described by her husband. He immediately called EMS, and they found the woman in ventricular fibrillation (arrhythmia). She was taken to a hospital where, fifteen minutes after admission, she was pronounced dead. This was the only information that I received with the body that was transferred from the hospital to Office of Medical Examiner.

The readers of my forensic stories might be surprised at how sparse our initial information about the deceased often is. "The dead body is talking," Doctor Spitz wrote in our forensic textbook. And indeed it is, but we have to be knowledgeable and very diligent to discern and interpret this talk. Our cases differ from one another, sometimes in a subtle way, and it is in the forensic pathologist's judgment to do whatever is necessary to open the secrets of the dead body.

It is early morning and this case is my first case of the day. Before starting the autopsy I would like to have more information about the deceased, but her relatives had not come yet, and there is no answer at the home telephone. It's busy all the time, either disconnected by the family stricken with disaster or busy with continuous calls from relatives and friends. Sometimes the relatives call us giving helpful information. But most frequently we talk with the family after the autopsy when they come for identification and expect to talk with us. Some of them are so shocked that they do not have the nerves for talking, and we patiently wait for the right time, understanding their pain.

On autopsy I saw a young Hispanic woman around age thirty of a normal height and light weight. Rigidity was present and libidity was fixed on the back; she had died the day before, and it was consistent with the story. She did not have signs of trauma, but she had signs of resuscitation that she received in the hospital on admission. There were bilateral intravenous lines on both forearms, signs of hospital intervention. After the external examination, I opened the body and all cavities, carefully studying all her organs. Her lungs were normal, and she did not have pulmonary embolism, the blood clots that could have moved from the deep vein of the lower extremities to the pulmonary arteries, causing sudden death. Her heart was of normal weight, and the coronary arteries had a normal pattern of distribution and were unremarkable. She did not have any congenital abnormalities, and the heart tissue was normal. All other organs including the brain did not show any abnormalities. The stomach contained a small amount of greenish fluid, and the small and large intestine were unremarkable except for the presence of liquid stool that I decided to send for bacteriology.

I saved her brain for study with a neuropathologist and submitted her blood for bacteriology to study and exclude infection or sepsis. I took for toxicology all the routine material for drugs, alcohol, and medication tests. I routinely submitted blood to the serology lab and sent small pieces of internal organs for microscopic study. All these were important steps, especially as I did not see anything abnormal during the autopsy. Multiple Kodachromes were taken of the body and organs. I made a decision to save the whole heart in case its study proved necessary.

As soon as I finished the autopsy, the husband and the sister of the deceased came for identification, and I had my time of talking with them. From the conversation, I learned that she had had a heart murmur from childhood, but otherwise "she did not have problems all her life." She had three children ages seven, twelve, and thirteen. The woman did not have a permanent doctor because she did not have any complaints. In the last two to three months, she had lost twenty pounds of her weight, though not intentionally, without any explanation. I informed the family that on autopsy I did not see an obvious reason for her death, that further studies would be done, and that I would contact them as soon as I finalized the case.

Soon after this conversation, I received a telephone call from the director of a family practice, who gave me very valuable information. The young woman had been under their care several years prior to her tragic death. In addition to regular gynecology care, an echogram had been done which revealed a mild mitral and tricuspid valve regurgitation (backflow of blood). The doctor did not know why the echogram was done, but after the echogram, the patient had been sent to a cardiologist. The director promised to find more information about the cardiologist, why the woman was sent to the cardiologist, and what more, if anything, had been done. She kept her promise, soon calling me with information that the patient had nine visits to the Bronx hospital, had been seen by the cardiologist and was scheduled for a pacemaker by the age of thirty to thirty-five (at the time, she was twenty-five). A few names of cardiologists were given to me, and I tried to reach them but with no success. But I was able to order the hospital chart through our medical investigator.

I received the results of the toxicology report that was negative for drugs, alcohol, and medication. Her brain was studied with a neuropathologist, and no abnormality was found. Microbiology of the blood and stool was negative. Multiple slides of internal organs, including many of the heart, did not reveal any abnormalities.

Soon I received a partial copy of the hospital chart with history of a couple of the patient's visits related to her gynecological care and her ECG, which had been taken at the age of twenty-six. I learned to interpret an ECG many years ago, as all medical doctors do, yet now it was not in the area of my expertise. All six pages of ECG, in addition to the charts, had interpretation comments: heart rate 42, A-V dissociation, **complete heart block** (abnormal conduction, arrhythmia). It was clear that something was wrong with the heart. I was lucky that I saved the whole heart after the autopsy.

I called the chief of pathology of the hospital, the cardio pathology expert. He was the editor of the cardiology journal and the author of many articles and a textbook in this field. I asked for the appointment and for permission to bring the heart of the deceased. As always, I received his permission to come immediately, and we did dissection of the heart, providing many more sections for microscopic study. We performed sections of the A-V node, which was not in the standard procedure during an autopsy. A block of tissue for a histology examination was obtained from the right atrium, near the coronary sinus. Also included with the sections were the tricuspid valve leaflet and the atrioventricular septum. The latter contained the A-V node immediately beneath the endocardium.

Grossly we did not see a tumor in this area, but the microscopic slides, which I rushed through our histology lab, revealed a cystic tumor of A-V node. This tumor was benign, consisted of multiple cystic spaces lined by several layers of blunt polygonal, mucin-producing cells. Detrimental was the location of the tumor that caused complete heart blockage, arrhythmia, and, finally, the sudden death of the young woman.

After this discovery, the chief of pathology immediately found one of the cardiologists, who four to five years before had seen this patient and requested an ECG, and all of us discussed the case. We learned from the cardiologist that the patient had had episodes of "heart racing" and occasional lightheadedness. The case was very revealing for all of us.

Complete congenital heart blockage has been recognized since 1846, yet the prognosis of the disease and management leaves a lot to be desired. In this case, a tumor could not be diagnosed when the patient was alive. It was so small that even after the autopsy, we found it only microscopically. But I also learned from this case that it was the right decision to save the whole heart—that gave me the opportunity to consult with the expert in this field. The family very often does not know and cannot provide the important information about certain conditions of their deceased relative. In cases of the sudden deaths of young people, it is important to talk with relatives and ask about such complaints as syncope, temporary loss of consciousness, episodes of "heart racing," and occasional lightheadedness, which could help us to think of and examine the hidden heart abnormalities.

The guidelines for prophylactic pacemaker implantation are not in the area of my expertise. According to medical literature, the development of these guidelines is a difficult issue due to the small number of patients and isolation of centers. This case tells us that there is room for improvement here as well.

HYPERTROPHIC CARDIOMYOPATHY

The death of a child is the worst devastating event, especially if the child dies unexpectedly, without any medical history. Unfortunately, it happens and is not so rare. Forensic pathologists get involved in these tragic cases. We feel a little better if the autopsy shows that the child's disease caused the unavoidable death and nothing could have been done to prevent it; at least in this case, the parents should not feel guilt in addition to the shocking event of the death itself. Here are two cases linked by a similarity of genetic origin.

Brian was a fifteen year old black teenager, tall, slim, and of normal weight, who lived with his parents and two younger siblings. He did not have significant medical history, except a history of asthma, a frequent companion in the poor families and neighborhoods. I really do not know with certainty why this is so. The only thing I feel is that the cases branded by asthma must be thoroughly examined and studied for the cause.

Brian was an average-grade student, loved sports, and had in every respect a typical teenager's behavior. Yet one day, during the school hours, he was found in the school yard unconscious and in cardiac arrest. Nobody saw how or why he collapsed. He was brought to a hospital by EMS. Resuscitation was continued in the hospital, but actually he was dead on arrival. He received Epinephrine, Atropine, Narcan, and D50, but nothing could help, and minutes after admission he was pronounced dead.

On autopsy there were no signs of any trauma. The only abnormal finding was a markedly enlarged heart weighing five hundred grams. The heart, however, did not show any congenital abnormality. So, the initial diagnosis was "pending further study." I had to see the results of toxicology for drugs, medication, and alcohol, and I needed a microscopic study of the heart and all other organs. I explained all this to Brian's mother, who was stricken by this tragedy.

The toxicology report came in ten days. There were no drugs, medication, or alcohol in the blood, but in the urine and bile, cannabinoids from marihuana were detected. Brian did not die because of drugs, but at some point he had used marihuana. By far the most significant finding was reported from a microscopic study of the heart. It discovered very strong changes in the heart tissue.

The heart itself and the microscopic report were consulted with our cardio-pathologist. She explained that microscopic sections from the heat showed disarray in muscle bundle arrangement. In some areas, the individual muscles were arranged in a haphazard manner with almost perpendicular orientation to each other. The small intra-myocardial vessels were thick, and the cardiac cells of the muscular tissue were enlarged.

The cause of death was hypertrophic cardiomyopathy.

***

Ian, a fourteen year old black teenager, had come from Alabama two weeks before and was a new student in his school. One day he suddenly collapsed in the music class in the school; he had seizures, and EMS was called. On arrival, EMS found that he showed no pulse. He was intubated and CPR was performed. On admission to the hospital, Ian's ECG was flat. He was re-intubated, and he received epinephrine, atropine, bicarbonate, and fluids. All attempts of resuscitation were unsuccessful, and twenty minutes after the admission he was pronounced dead with the cause: cardiac arrest. There was no history of either trauma or drug use.

On autopsy, the body was a well-developed male appearing to be consistent with the stated age of fourteen, measuring five feet, five inches, and weighing one hundred and twenty-five pounds. There was nothing abnormal in the skull and brain, except a two centimeter bleeding of the soft tissue of the left side of the skull, obviously resulting from a final fall when the boy collapsed. All organs were absolutely normal. But the heart had a predominant left ventricular enlargement. There was no congenital abnormality. A section of the heart was taken for the microscopic study. The cause of death was preliminarily put as "pending further study."

In two weeks, I received the toxicology report—no drugs, alcohol, or medication in the system. The brain was studied by our neuropathologist, and no pathology was observed. All other organs did not have any disease. However, the microscopy of the heart showed significant muscle disorganization. The case was also consulted with our cardio-pathologist. I called the parents and explained to them the cause of death.

***

Both cases are examples of the so called idiopathic cardiac hypertrophy (the enlargement or overgrowth of the heart or its constituent cells). Over the last decade significant advancements have been made in understanding the clinical and genetic basis of sudden cardiac death in youngsters. It is a genetic cardiac disorder caused by mutations in at least one of the protein genes, which can lead to both structural and arrhythmic abnormalities. The families are in shock losing otherwise healthy youngsters. This tragic event presents a challenge for the clinicians involved in management of the surviving family members. They must be seen and evaluated by a cardiologist, a geneticist, and a psychologist.

INSIDIOUS CHILDREN'S DISEASE

One of my three cases after the triage that day was a case of a twelve year old girl, Sabrina, who was admitted to the hospital in cardiac arrest and, in spite of all resuscitation measures, was pronounced dead shortly after admission.

As usually, we started from obtaining and studying all available information prior to performing the autopsy. Upon receiving this case from the hospital, the medical investigator had contacted the hospital and received everything they had to share with us.

The day before, the child had complained to her mother of abdominal pain and vomiting and had been taken to the hospital's ER for evaluation. The girl had been having fever, cough, and a runny nose for the past two weeks. In the hospital she was diagnosed with gastritis and after four hours was discharged home. But she continued feeling not well after the discharge. The mother, trying to comfort her, gave her soup and put her to bed. At around 2:00 am the mother woke up to check on her daughter and found her unresponsive on the bathroom floor. She called 911. EMS responded to her residence and started resuscitation, intubated the girl, inserted IV lines and administered Narcan due to pinpoint pupils (nowadays narcotics are big concern). The girl was taken to the hospital, this time a different one, where resuscitation in the ER continued for nearly two hours, until she was pronounced dead.

Children usually do not die of myocardial infarct, pulmonary embolism, or brain aneurism rupture as adults do. So, it I thought it might be either acute myocarditis, considering the history of the viral infection in the last two weeks, or an acute abdomen, considering abdominal pain and vomiting, the complaints that initially brought the child to the hospital. Teenagers, much better than small children, could differentiate the localization of their pain. The child did have a history of aortic and mitral valve insufficiency, but the hospital doctor did not believe that cardiac history contributed to her death. With all that, the cause of death was not clear to the hospital, and the case was reported to the Office of Medical Examiner.

On the table of the autopsy room, I found the body of the twelve year old Hispanic girl, five feet, six inches tall and weighing one hundred and thirty pounds. There were no signs of trauma, except the resuscitation marks on the chest and intravenous lines of the wrists. The internal investigation showed all organs in their anatomically normal position. Yet her heart was enlarged, considering her age and weight. There was nothing wrong in the abdominal cavity. I did not see anything wrong with the brain. So, it became clear that it was not an acute abdomen, and there was no bleeding in the brain. Thus, I thought, the heart should resolve the cause of her sudden death. Acute myocarditis? We would see. Of course as usual, I was taking specimens for a toxicological study, but I really did not suspect drugs.

That day I put, as a cause of her death, "pending further study," and I released her body. I planned to study small pieces of her internal organs under the microscope, receive the toxicology report as our routine procedure, look through her heart with our cardio-pathologist, talk with the parents for more details of the girl's health, and find more information from the cardiologist who had seen her before.

I called the girl's mother, and a very somber Hispanic female answered my call. I expressed to her my condolences, but she wanted to speak in Spanish. I promised to get back to her after I found our Spanish-speaking secretary. Meanwhile, our office clerk informed me that the father of the deceased had come for identification and would like to speak with me. In the ID room I found a young Hispanic male with dark glasses. Unfortunately, he did not know much about the recent events because he did not live with the family, but he told me that his daughter had been an absolutely healthy girl and that her mother had taken her to the hospital because she had abdominal pain. I explained to him my preliminary findings and the steps of the further examination and investigation.

From Sabrina's mother, I found the name and the telephone number of the cardiologist who had seen her daughter and had mentioned "very mild heart problems." I promised to contact the mother as soon as I finalized the cause of her daughter's death.

My next call was to the cardiologist. After trying four different numbers, dialing the different offices and hospitals, I finally found him, but he did not remember the girl and could not immediately find information because he was at a different location from where he kept his records. The cardiologist promised to call me back the next day.

The next day I received a telephone call from the chief of the pediatric department where the girl was initially admitted. She wanted to know the result of the autopsy. I informed her about my strong suspicion of acute myocarditis, considering the absence of any findings except the enlarged heart. The doctor mentioned to me the important fact that the x-ray made in the hospital showed that Sabrina had cardiomegaly (an enlarged heart). The pediatrician was obviously upset. No wonder—it was a very sad case of the child's death, especially after they had initially released the girl home.

Then again, I called the girl's cardiologist and learned that he had seen her one year ago because of a heart murmur found by the pediatrician, but nothing serious was confirmed, and he thought about very mild aortic and mitral insufficiency.

An unexpected call came from the nurse of an agency studying an adverse vaccine reaction. She informed me that, one week before her death, Sabrina had received vaccination for Varicella, Hepatitis A, and Cardisil (human papilloma virus). That was important information. I thought, "How could they administer these vaccinations if she had a viral infection, or did she get these clinical symptoms after the vaccinations?"

As I expected, I received from our cardio-pathologist the report with the diagnosis: myocarditis of probable viral etiology. The toxicology lab did not find anything unusual; virology and bacteriology results were negative.

Myocarditis is an inflammatory disease of the myocardium (cardiac muscles) associated with cardiac dysfunction. Variable clinical manifestations are present, from latent to very severe clinical forms such as acute congestive heart failure and sudden death. Early and definite diagnosis still depends on the detection of inflammatory infiltrates in the endometrial biopsy specimens. The optimum treatment for myocarditis in children is unknown, and the treatment is supportive, if the diagnosis is made.

I called the mother, as I had promised, and explained to her the cause of the child's death. She was furious with the hospital that initially sent the child home.

I called the hospital's chief of pediatrics, and we discussed the diagnosis and their clinical data. Retrospectively, an ECG could have been helpful. Cardiac enzymes, tachycardia (rapid pulse), and cardiomegaly—all together should have helped to diagnose myocarditis and given reason to put the child in the hospital for observation and supportive therapy. The case would be definitely discussed on the medical conference.

I contacted the agency studying the adverse reaction of the vaccination and informed them about the final diagnosis. I was assured by the nurse with whom I initially discussed the case that the government very seriously studies the adverse results of vaccination. For the time being, she did not have any data suggesting the cause relationship between vaccination and myocarditis.

***

She was a beautiful, tall, third grade girl, one of the best students in her class. Maritza did not miss one day in her school year. She participated in many activities including soft ball and modern dancing. Her two younger brothers followed her and copied in everything that their big sister did. But for the last four days Maritza had had a severe cough that did not stop her attending the school and participating in the Tuesday dance class. Of course, she did not feel the usual strength, but children do have that quality of continuing to do what they like. Children's energy gives them extra strength that adults would not have.

Maritza's condition drastically worsened, and she developed shortness of breath. Her mother, a bronchial asthma patient all her life, tried to help her daughter with her Albuterol pump, but there was no improvement. When the mother found the girl unresponsive, she called emergency workers, and Maritza was admitted to the hospital. On admission the girl was very pale, with no signs of respiration or pulse. In spite of all resuscitation efforts, Maritza was pronounced dead forty minutes after admission. The child had not had any medical problems before this admission. The family requested an autopsy, and the body was sent to the Office of Medical Examiner.

On the next day I performed the autopsy of this child. As always, according to our routine procedures of children's autopsies, x-ray of the whole body was done to exclude trauma. Also, multiple photos of the body were taken; swabs of the mouth, vagina, and anus were done for exclusion of any sexual assault. The girl was of normal height and weight. She did not have any sign of trauma. Her lungs were edematous, full of fluid, but that often happens and by itself is not indicative of the cause. The heart of the deceased was of normal weight and grossly normal appearance. She did not have any congenital abnormalities, and her internal organs looked normal. I took small pieces of the internal organs for a microscopic study. I submitted her blood for a microbiology study and took everything that was necessary for a toxicology study.

My diagnosis after the autopsy was "pending further study," because I really did not know why the child died. But I did know for sure that she did not have any trauma as a cause of her death.

After the autopsy, I received a call from Maritza's father. I explained to him my preliminary findings and the necessity for continuation of the study. The father was very upset. Removal of two other children from the home by a social worker was only aggravating their disaster. These two children had been taken to the hospital, checked, and pronounced healthy, and in spite of that, they had been held away from the family. I immediately called the detective who was on this case, but he was not on duty at that time. I called the social worker involved with the case, but I could not reach her either. I called her supervisor and discussed the case with him, and he gave me the telephone number of another supervisor in a higher position. I called this other supervisor who kindly helped me find the social worker on the case. She confirmed that the children were taken from the parents following the instructions on how to handle the situation in the case of a child's death. The children had been temporary placed with their grandmother. I wanted to talk with the district attorney who handled the case, but the social worker did not know who the district attorney was. "Why did the mother give the child the inhalator?" she asked me. She also told me that she would not release the children until the "pending" diagnosis changed to final. So I did the only thing left available to me—I immediately called our first deputy and rushed the case.

A microscopic study of the heart gave the answer to the puzzle. Maritza had granulomatous giant cell myocarditis, probably of viral etiology. All other studies—toxicology, brain study, microbiology, and serology were negative.

I called and talked with the chief of microbiology because microbiology was negative in the blood and in the pleural fluid that I sent to them. I called and talked with the chief of virusology lab, but I found that they did not do viral studies postmortem (that is, after death). I called the virusology lab in Albany, and they referred me to their virusologist who, in turn, informed me that they did not do postmortem viral studies, either. He suggested that the enterovirus was most probably the cause of the granulomatous myocarditis. I called the father, expressed my condolences again and explained the cause of his daughter's death. Shortly after, the other children were returned to the parents.

Idiopathic (not of a clear cause) giant cell myocarditis is a rare but frequently fatal disorder. Patients usually die of heart failure and ventricular arrhythmia unless a cardiac transplantation is performed. Transplantation is the treatment of choice for most patients. Maritza had neither that option nor the time for it.

During my career as a forensic pathologist, I had several cases of the children's acute myocarditis. All of them had a history of a few days of "cold" followed by the rapid deterioration and death. There was no time for diagnostics, endometrial biopsy, or cardiac transplant. I think that our medicine is still far from perfect in diagnostics and treatment of this insidious fatal disease. Of course, the important requirement to the proper diagnosis is the physician's awareness, quick response, immediate hospitalization, and supportive treatment.

SICKLE CELL DISORDER

This baby girl was found unresponsive by her father in the crib. She had had a fever the night before, and the mother had given her Tylenol. The mother was age thirty-eight, and the father, age forty, both carried sickle cell trait. But baby Rosa had sickle cell anemia. During her entire thirteen months of life, Rosa was susceptible to respiratory infection. Also I learned that there were two other siblings in the family, ages eight and twenty.

Rosa was seen alive for the last time around 6:00 am, when the mother went to check on her and again gave her Tylenol. Sometimes afterwards, the worried father went to the bedroom to see the child and found her unresponsive. He immediately started CPR, and they called 911. Rosa was brought to the hospital by EMS in the state of cardiac arrest. Chest compression and ventilation were applied. On arrival her temperature was ninety-eight point three. In the hospital she was intubated, and all the protocol of resuscitation was followed, but nothing helped, and she was pronounced dead. There was no sign of trauma, and the only physical finding on external examination was an enlarged spleen. A cerebrospinal tap was performed, a blood culture was taken, and the results were pending from the hospital lab. But hemoglobin and hematocrit (the volume percentage of erythrocytes in the whole blood) tests were not done because there was not enough blood. The child was actually dead on arrival. The hospital reported the case to the Office of Medical Examiner because the cause of death was unknown, and the child died in a short period of time.

Before I started the autopsy, I called and talked with the hospital pediatrician. When the doctor had last seen her one month earlier, Rosa did not have anemia. She was "okay," but her hematocrit was a little low. Then, Rosa's father called me, adding that they, the mother and the father, had sickle cell trait, but that the child had sickle cell disease. The hospital later confirmed that the child had sickle cell disease. All these abnormalities are genetically transmitted and characterized by abnormal hemoglobin, some of which may result in anemia. This disease is considered milder than other forms of hemoglobinopathy (defective hemoglobin synthesis).

The father also described to me the child's condition when he discovered her in the crib, "She was gasping for air!" He obviously was in a lot of pain, and my heart was going out to him. A child's death is the worst tragedy.

On external examination I did not find anything abnormal. The child was of normal height and weight, without any signs of trauma. There were signs of therapeutic intervention: a tube in the mouth, intravenous marks on the left forearm and on both lower extremities. Internal examination grossly revealed that all organs were of the normal size and weight, except the spleen. The spleen was enlarged and had the marked red-bluish appearance on the surface of the cut. It definitely looked abnormal.

Our photographer took a lot of pictures. I took small pieces of internal organs for microscopic studies and sent material for microbiology and virus studies. Blood was sent to the serology lab with a request to do hemoglobin, hematocrit, and also hemoglobin electrophoresis. The latter was done because the child had sickle cell disease. The abnormal hemoglobin is distinguished by electrophoretic mobility and has been designated by letters. As we do routinely, I sent material for the toxicology lab. I took blood and bile for a genetic study. Now I had to wait for all these studies to make my final diagnosis. I called the father and explained my preliminary findings and the studies that would follow. Of course, the body was immediately released with the temporary diagnosis "pending further study." I promised the father to call him immediately after I got everything done to make the final diagnosis.

Our laboratories did their job promptly, and within a month I received everything to finalize the case. While waiting for the reports, I had studied medical literature for interpretation of the findings. The toxicology laboratory did not find any drugs or medication. From the serology laboratory I received the result of the hemoglobin electrophoresis, suggesting the type of disease S-C, similar to the hospital information. The brain and spinal cord study did not reveal abnormalities.

Microscopic slides of all internal organs were done. The heart slides showed immature blood cells in the small blood vessels, and immature blood cells were found in lungs. The larynx had focal areas of inflammation that suggested the respiratory (probably viral) infection. Liver slides showed sickle cells (crescent-shaped) and compensatory activity of the liver. Kidney slides also had sickle cells. And of course the spleen, the organ that looked so abnormal during the autopsy, was packed with sickle cells that completely replaced the white pulp of the spleen.

So, I made the diagnosis: sickle cell disease (S-C) with spleen sequestration (physiological separation).

In spite of many years experience in general and forensic pathology, this case was the first time I had seen spleen sequestration. I decided to get a consultation in the New York University hospital. I went to the chief of pediatric pathology, a very experienced and highly qualified doctor. She also did not recall seeing this kind of the case, and she invited the hematologist of NYU. All three of us discussed and agreed with the diagnosis. I called the family and explained to them the cause of the child's death. Unfortunately, it could not bring their child back.

A study of natural history of sickle cell hemoglobinopathy was initiated in 1978–1979. Most of previous studies of death due to these diseases were performed retrospectively on a small number of patients. The direct cause of death for ages one to three was infection. Central nervous system complications in young patients also cause severe disability and death. Children with sickle cell anemia and its variants have much higher risk for sudden death due to sepsis.

The thirteen month old Rosa had an acute spleen sequestration crisis that was characterized by sudden trapping of blood within the spleen, increased spleen size, a drop in hemoglobin concentration, and an abnormally decreased volume of the circulating fluid in the body, which may lead to shock and even death. The adults with sickle cell hemoglobinopathy suffer mostly from multiple spleen infarctions resulting in fibrosis (scarring) of the spleen. In all cases, the clinical features vary from fatigue, fever, vomiting, abdominal pain, and difficulties in breathing to the severe fatal shock—exactly what this child had. The death might have been preventable had the child been immediately brought to a hospital where pediatric hematologists have developed protocols for the evaluation and treatment of febrile children with sickle cell disorder. The need for parental education and counseling about this illness and its complications could not be over emphasized.

***

Five years after the death of the child with spleen sequestration caused by sickle cell disease, I had a similar case of a young black woman of age twenty-seven. According to her family, she had been a healthy woman with no history of previous diseases, full of life, a lover of chorus singing in the church. But after a short trip to Detroit followed by a respiratory infection, she had not felt well. Her weakness became so severe that she even could not participate in her routine church singing. She went to a hospital with breathing problems. Six hours after the admission, she suddenly developed cardiac-respiratory arrest and died. Before starting the autopsy, I called and talked with the hospital physician who gave me information about her breathing problems, recent respiratory infection, yellow eyes, absence of alcohol and drug usage, fever, and very low platelets in the blood. She was very dehydrated on admission. Because of the death shortly after the admission and also because of the unknown cause of death, the body was sent to us.

On autopsy her liver was enlarged, and she had a huge spleen, five to six times larger than normal, with the same characteristic dark red color that I had already seen before in the above described case. "Is it a case of the sequestrated spleen?" I immediately thought. I ordered, in addition to our routine studies, the hemoglobin study by our serology lab. And I again talked with the family after the autopsy, giving them my preliminary result and asking if she had sickle cell disease. The answer was "No, she did not have it," and other members of her family did not have it, either.

I ordered and received more information from the hospital, and learned that she had a negative test for hepatitis, and her blood culture was negative. She had a low platelet count and very low hemoglobin and hematocrit.

Microscopic study of the internal organs showed... sickle cells, and the spleen appeared packed with sickle cells—very similar to the above child's case. And sickle cell disease mutation analysis of the postmortem blood done by our serology lab came with the following result: positive for one copy of the Hemoglobin S mutation and negative for the Hemoglobin C mutation. Therefore, she was at least a carrier of sickle cell anemia.

I discussed the case with the deputy, then went to NYU and discussed the case with their hematologist, who immediately agreed with my interpretation. I put the cause of death: sequestration crisis with anemia and splenomegaly (enlarged spleen) in patient with S sickle cell trait.

I think in this case, as in the case of the child, the respiratory infection provoked the sequestration crisis with sudden death. I discussed the case with the family and advised them to check themselves for sickle cell disease or the trait.

***

The question arises if the sickle cell trait should be considered asymptomatic or as a benign condition during physical activity.

"New York City has temporary suspended its physical examination for firefighters after the death of an applicant who collapsed after taking the grueling test at the New York Coliseum," reported one of the New York newspapers.

Back in late 1980s, in the spring, after taking the vigorous physical exam, eight candidates were taken to the hospital because of the ill effect after this test. But the main reason for suspension of this test was the death of one of them, a young man in his early twenties. It was a very public case from the beginning because of the importance of the testing for the fire fighters whose strenuous work required the recruits to be in the excellent shape. Only five thousand of the twenty-nine thousand potential firefighters have passed this demanding test of strength and overall fitness. I really did not know that the firefighter job was so popular in New York. It was a dangerous kind of profession, and I always looked at them with admiration—tall and strong men in their "Martian" uniform, as they were. My respect to them was grandiose. And after the September 11, I added a very sentimental feeling for them, especially for my neighbors—the Ladder 13, who lost nine people that sad day.

But back to the case, I was assigned to it in the early morning. A twenty-four year old young man collapsed during the physical test at the New York Coliseum. I received the following information: The young man after the test did not feel well and complained of back pain, muscle pain, and severe weakness. He felt dehydrated, having dry mucous membranes. He was taken to the hospital; his ECG revealed arrhythmia, his potassium was very high and continued rising despite the therapy. The specific skeletal muscle enzyme was elevated. His urine contained blood, and urine output was very low despite receiving extra fluid. The clinical picture was consistent with high potassium in the blood secondary to massive muscle injury from rhabdomyolysis (disintegration of muscles) with subsequent cardiac arrest. Six hours after admission, he was pronounced dead in spite of the treatment.

From the hospital, I received information that the deceased had a history of asthma and sickle cell trait. The autopsy did not reveal anything unusual. All his internal organs were of normal size, weight, and appearance. The toxicology report came back negative for drugs and positive for small amount of medication given to him in the hospital. But microscopic slides did reveal sickle cell erythrocytes in all organs. Slides of the muscles showed areas of acute rhabdomyolysis.

I went with all his information and slides to the NYU hospital and consulted the case with their leading nephro-pathologist, who, however, was a little skeptical about observing sickle cells in the formalin fixed slides. But our neuropathologist did not have problems seeing and admitting the sickle cell erythrocytes in the blood vessels and changes in muscles. In addition, I sent all material for consultation to my former boss in a Michigan hospital, where I did my residency in pathology, a known and very knowledgeable nephro-pathologist. His conclusion was that the young man did have acute changes in the muscles, and he did see sickle cells in the formalin fixed tissue, the latter being consistent with the history of sickle cell disorder.

After all studies and consultations, I put the diagnosis: hyperkalemia (increase of potassium) and acute renal failure followed strenuous exercise. Exertional rhabdomyolisis. Sickle cell trait.

Of course, I studied the medical literature for information on this subject. I learned that between 1970–1974, at two large military installations, among thousands of trainees who were subjected to the strong physical and environmental stresses, only four recruits were hospitalized because of acute disintegration of muscles due to physical exertion, renal failure, and disorders of blood clotting. The illness followed the performance of vigorous exercise. These four patients had sickle cell trait. In more recent literature, I found more descriptions of complications and even sudden deaths in military recruits, affected by sickle cell trait, during extensive exercise, although the sickle cell trait is usually considered as a benign and innocuous carrier state, rather than a disease.

The question arises if more selective consideration must be done in choosing recruits with sickle cell trait for duty and professions subjected to vigorous exercise.

ACUTE EPIGLOTTITIS

My first encounter with the sudden death due to acute epiglottitis was in the Manhattan office in early 1990s. A forty-five year old woman came to the hospital complaining of sore throat. While waiting in the admission room of the hospital for a few hours, she developed respiratory arrest, and, in spite of all resuscitation efforts, succumbed to death. This became our case because the deceased was in the hospital for very short period of time. The hospital did not have a diagnosis, and cardio-respiratory arrest as a clinical cause does not provide a sufficient explanation—most people finally die because of cardio-respiratory arrest.

I performed the autopsy on this relatively young woman and did not find anything except acute inflammation of the epiglottis that was cherry red, stiff, and swollen. The epiglottis is the cartilaginous structure that overhangs the entrance to the larynx and serves to prevent the swallowed food from entering the larynx and trachea. The post-autopsy histological study confirmed the acute inflammation of the epiglottis. Postmortem bacteriology was negative. The toxicology study for drugs and medication were also negative.

The cause of death was issued: acute epiglottitis. Manner of death: natural.

A few years after this, I had another case that immediately reminded me of the first one. A forty year old woman was admitted to the ICU with respiratory arrest. She was transported from home by EMS. She lived with her family in a shared apartment, and on the night of presentation she complained, "I can't breathe." The family called 911, and EMS responded. Upon admission to the ER, the woman was found unresponsive. She was placed on ventilator support, but after three days in ICU the woman was pronounced dead. The family requested an autopsy. According to information received from the family, she had been in an unusual state of health prior to reporting to work, coughing in the bathroom at work, with her eyes very watery. She had stated, "My throat don't feel right." She had decided to go from her work to a hospital, where the medical staff informed her that she had a sore throat and instructed her to take a throat lozenge. She returned home but her condition was only worsening, eventually leading to the respiratory arrest and the call to EMS. This case was accepted by the Office of Medical Examiner.

The next day I performed the autopsy. The body was of normal height and weight without any signs of trauma, showing only hospital signs of intervention: resuscitation marks and intravenous marks and lines. Her all internal organs were normal. The only abnormal thing was a markedly red epiglottis. I took her blood and spinal fluid for microbiology, all necessary material for histology and also for toxicology tests on drugs and medication. I already knew that a test for drugs was performed in the hospital, and it was negative. The bacteriology result in her blood was negative (she received antibiotics during three days of hospitalization). The test of spinal fluid revealed Staphylococcus epidermidis, but I could ignore that because it might be a contamination—this microbe is normally present on the skin surface.

The histology test confirmed the diagnosis: acute epiglottitis.

From my conversation with the hospital physician, I learned that the first time the woman came to the hospital with shortness of breath and a sore throat they did not manage to evaluate her because she left the hospital. When she was admitted for the second time, she already was in cardiac arrest, and EMS had trouble intubating her (probably because of the swollen and stiff epiglottis). In the emergency room they did intubate her, noticing the swollen local cord. But she was already brain dead, and her blood culture grew nothing

Both cases presented a rapidly progressing infection and inflammation of the epiglottis and surrounding tissue. It leads to sudden respiratory obstruction and death.

As a former pediatrician, I was familiar and aware of this very dangerous disease in children that required immediate hospitalization. Direct visualization of the epiglottis is the diagnostic. Because the sudden and complete airway obstruction could be expected, a continually adequate airway must be secured immediately. Speed of action is vital.

The incidence in children has dramatically declined in the past decade due to widespread vaccination. H-Influenza type was the most common cause before the vaccination. But currently, other organisms might become a cause of this dangerous disease. Acute epiglottitis among adults is on the rise, according to the medical literature, and my two cases were the evidence to that.

Soon after I performed the last autopsy, I myself had an acute laryngitis with sore throat, hoarseness, and a little fever. Remembering these two cases, I, who not for the first time had such laryngitis, started to develop difficulties with breathing, sweating, trembling, and fear of dying. Probably it was a panic attack, but I immediately asked my husband to bring me to the nearby hospital, instructing him to tell them of what I was afraid (acute epiglottitis with airway obstruction). I instructed my husband not to allow the hospital personnel to spend the precious time for paperwork, an ECG, and other tests that would show normal anyway, at least in my opinion. I was in a panic, breathing heavily and very often. My husband somehow managed to scare the otherwise unshakable personnel, and I was given oxygen right away and was told that the otolaryngologist would come as soon as possible. He indeed came, confirmed the swelling of epiglottis and vocal cord, and checked my larynx. I did not have a drastic fatal situation, and after two hours of observation was discharged with suggestions for treatment. The diagnosis was acute laryngitis, and my insurance denied the charges.

Well, I was alive. I could have fought with the insurance company, but I did not.

COCAINE "MULE"

In the mid-1990s, in the Bronx, a park employee found the body of unknown man wrapped in a rug. The police were called, and the body was sent to the Office of Medical Examiners. I received the case.

The body was slightly decomposed with fixed libidity at the front and absent rigidity. The man had gray trousers, a blue shirt, yellow underwear, and gray socks. There was no ID or any other documents for that matter. X-ray of the whole body was taken for two reasons: exclusion of gunshot wounds and identification of the body. Even though externally I did not see any gunshot wounds, the bullets from possible old gunshot wounds might still be in the body. X-ray did not reveal any bullets. There was nothing unusual on external examination, except the presence of scars and needle marks on the forearm areas, which suggested that the deceased was a chronic drug user.

Initial examination of the skull and brain revealed bleeding of the soft vascular membrane of the cerebellum and both hemispheres. It could be explained by decomposition of the body, but could be real as well. The internal organs showed no abnormalities, except signs of decomposition, but the big surprise was in the stomach. The stomach contained six balloon capsules with whitish powder. I looked at my technician, who was in deep thought, yet by that time was diligently opening the small and the large intestines in the big bucket filled with water. I could not believe my eyes—multiple balloon capsules were floating in the water, but Ann, my technician, did not show any surprise upon viewing the unusual contents.

We counted all these capsules—one hundred and two! They weighed twelve hundred grams. Our photographer took all necessary pictures, and evidence immediately took the capsules away. I put the cause of death "pending further study" because I needed to see the toxicology results.

In about a month, I received the results of the toxicology tests. The deceased's blood had 7.0 mg/l of cocaine; in the gastric contents there was 99 mg/kg of cocaine; and the content of balloons was determined as cocaine. These were very high numbers indeed, but actually both numbers by themselves were not that important because cocaine and opiates do not have specific toxic levels under which they are safe—every amount and level could cause death. There were cases in our practice when a very low level, such as 0.1 mg/l, caused the death of young and athletic people. They did not die because of overdose; they died mainly because of cardiac arrhythmia. The relatives of the deceased often asked us about the level of drugs in the blood, "Is it a lot?" And we, over and over again, would explain that any level of these drugs could cause the death.

The final cause of death was acute cocaine intoxication. Manner of death: accidental. The identification of the deceased never was made because nobody claimed the body.

This was a case of a "mule" transporting the packages of narcotics within his gastro-intestinal tract and dying because of acute intoxication due to the bursting of one or more packages. This was my first case of this "modern life" problem. I had few more cases, but, as I learned from an article written in 2004 by a colleague, in our office we had fifty cases of heroine and cocaine mules from 1990 to 2001. Alternatively, one Pennsylvania medical examiner reported the first case of a mule in 2005. Obviously, New York has much more of these arriving traffickers because New York was and is the destination of millions of visitors and tourists every day, and many of them are from the drug-producing countries. Body packing should be suspected in anyone with signs of drug-induced toxic effects upon arrival at the city terminal. Body packing of illegal drugs has increased in the last decades due to increased drug trafficking in other countries. More and more countries are reporting the increase of this practice: France, Italy, Poland, Ireland, Germany, England, Iran, Spain, and Israel.

In the older reports the body packers were young man, usually chronic drug abusers. But the demography of this group has changed, and children, older people, and even pregnant women get involved in this illegal business. The idea is evacuation of the capsules through the natural way, but it does not always happen this way, and clinical outcome of the body packer is unpredictable. Acute drug intoxication after rupture or leaking of the drug capsules causes cardio-respiratory arrest, psychosis, and convulsions. Another outcome is intestinal obstruction, sometimes with perforation, requiring immediate surgery.

The body packers' action is illegal and criminal, but the mules probably do not realize how dangerous the presence of the capsules in their bodies is. Body packers usually die unknown because the people involved in this transaction do not care about them. They do not call for medical help when a body packer develops signs of acute drug intoxication and it is still possible to help. When body packers die, their bodies are dumped without identification. The world of drug dealers is ruthless.

PYTHON

On the evening news I heard about very unusual case: a python killed his owner. Sacrificing my usual early morning ballet exercise, I decided to go to work earlier then my colleague, so I could choose the case. It turned out not to be necessary because my colleague, a young and eager doctor, had arrived before me anyway and already had the cases distributed, giving the python case to me. I was lucky!

Just as I was prepared to go to morgue, I received a frantic call from a Mr. Boos, "Are you a forensic pathologist?" he asked.

"Yes, I am "

"So, you are a Quincy!" (The famous TV character I first saw sometimes in 1980s).

"I want to tell you," went on he, "that this snake could never ever kill anybody. My daughter was raised with the python that slept with her in the same bed. Yes, I know their kind very well. In fact, I even wrote a book, *The Snakes of Guava*, back in 1969 or 1970. Unfortunately, it was never published. No, I did not receive any formal education, but I was from the family where two of us (my father and my brother) were members of the National Geographic Society. By the way, in addition to a python, I have two other snakes, one alligator, five cats, one dog, one wife, and one daughter. Yes, I have enough space; I am living in Greenwich Village and have a house. The python they had on the news was a baby comparatively to mine. I am telling you, look for murder—somebody killed the man!"

Then I received a telephone call from mother of the deceased.

She expressed hesitation about necessity of the autopsy, "I know that he died because of this snake, but people raise my doubts."

I explained to her why it is necessary to do the autopsy. We did not know why her boy was dead.

"He was a clean good boy. He loved these snakes very much. All the money that I gave him, he spent on snakes."

I am pathologist of many years, but I still painfully react on seeing young and presumably healthy people dead. This young snake-loving man was a nineteen-year-old, muscular, good-looking black man. On external examination he had very few petechias (small pinpoint bleeding of the sclera and conjunctivae). We are always looking for these non-specific signs of asphyxia. He did not have any marks on his neck or chest. The only unusual finding was the appearance of his right third finger—the nail was bent upside down. The deceased also had signs of therapeutic intervention: a tube in the mouth, intravenous marks, and pads for ECG.

Internal examination revealed areas of the neck muscles and fascia (a sheet of fibrous tissue beneath the surface of the skin) bleeding. There were no fractures; there were edema (an excessive accumulation of serous fluid in the tissue) and congestion of the lungs (excessive blood accumulation), nonspecific findings in many autopsies.

I put the temporary diagnosis as "pending further study" because I decided to wait for the toxicology study of medication, illegal drugs, and alcohol in the blood, urine, and bile. I would also examine under the microscope the slides of the internal organs to exclude the possibility of a disease that could cause the young man's death. I again called the mother of the deceased and explained to her the need for additional studies, and I released the body for funeral. I promise to call her as soon as I received the results.

Meanwhile, the newspapers gave me a lot of information about the snakes. A snake expert said that, contrary to popular belief, the pythons cannot be trained—they do not really learn to respond to people's commands or recognize them. They operate on instinct. Pythons are not poisonous and do not generally attack people. Yet a human might have a scent from an animal on the hands, and the instinct of the snake might take over. Pythons are incredibly strong. This Burmese python, bought for $300 three months before at a Pet City store, was about twelve feet long with weight of forty-five pounds! Pythons kill their prey by coiling around the victim and squeezing the life out of it. They are fed on small mammals like rabbits and guineas pigs. They also have been known to eat small deer, monkeys, and even jackals. They generally avoid humans. But there have been reports of killer snakes. In 1993, an eighty pound python asphyxiated a Colorado teenager. A year earlier, a twenty-eight year old snake lover from Toronto had been squeezed to death by his pet python.

Microscopic study of the internal organs did not reveal anything wrong with the young man. Toxicology studies were also negative: no drugs, no medication, and no alcohol. He was clean. Police investigators, after talking with his mother and friends, gave me some more details. The young man very often kept the python around his neck. He had bought a chicken to feed the python, and the snake might have moved abruptly toward the chicken meat on the floor, thus squeezing the young man's neck. That could explain the bent fingernail if the young man tried to release the neck pressure that caused his death.

I put the final diagnosis: asphyxia due to pressure to neck by python. The manner of death: accidental.

After I talked with the mother of the deceased, I called Mr. Boos who had doubts about the ability of a python to cause the death. There was no answer. I hope he is still alive and has read the newspaper information about pythons.

In Central Park, I sometimes see young men with snakes around their necks and curious crowds of adults and children around trying to touch the "pet." Sometimes I try to share with them my sad experience about the killer python, yet nobody takes me seriously.